A Research Portfolio o
Chronic Fatigue

Edited by Robin Fox

for the Linbury Trust

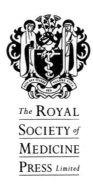

The ROYAL
SOCIETY *of*
MEDICINE
PRESS *Limited*

©1998 Royal Society of Medicine Press Limited
1 Wimpole Street, London W1M 8AE, UK
16 East 69th Street, New York NY 10021, USA

British Library Cataloguing in Publication Data

A catalogue record for this book is available from the British Library

ISBN 1-85315-367-2

Typeset by Dobbie Typesetting Limited, Tavistock, Devon
Printed in Great Britain by Ebenezer Baylis, The Trinity Press, Worcester

CONTENTS

CONTRIBUTORS

Professor Louis Appleby, *Department of Psychiatry, University of Manchester*

Dr Phillip Cash, *Department of Medical Microbiology, University of Aberdeen*

Trudie Chalder, *Department of Psychological Medicine, King's College School of Medicine and Dentistry, London*

Dr Anthony J Cleare, *Department of Psychological Medicine, King's College School of Medicine and Dentistry, London*

Dr GB Clements, *Regional Virus Laboratory, Gartnavel General Hospital, Glasgow*

Dr Helen Cope, *Wellcome Trust, London*

Professor Anthony S David, *Institute of Psychiatry, London*

Professor Timothy G Dinan, *Department of Psychiatry, Royal College of Surgeons in Ireland, Dublin*

Dr Robin Fox, *Journal of the Royal Society of Medicine, Royal Society of Medicine, London*

Dr Beatriz Gimenez, *Department of Molecular and Cell Biology, University of Aberdeen*

Professor Malcolm Jackson, *Department of Medicine, University of Liverpool*

Dr Eileen Joyce, *Department of Psychiatry, Imperial College School of Medicine, London*

Dr Anne McArdle, *Department of Medicine, University of Liverpool*

Dr Lucinda V Scott, *Department of Psychiatry, Trinity College Medical School, Dublin*

Dr Michael Sharpe, *Department of Psychiatry, University of Edinburgh*

Dr Jim Waterhouse, *Diabetes and Endocrinology Research Group, University Hospital Aintree, Liverpool*

Mrs Alison Wearden, *Department of Clinical Psychology, University of Manchester*

Professor Simon Wessely, *CFS Research Unit, King's College School of Medicine and Dentistry, London*

Dr Peter White, *Department of Psychological Medicine, St Bartholomew's and the Royal London School of Medicine and Dentistry, London*

Professor Gareth Williams, *Diabetes and Endocrinology Research Group, University Hospital Aintree, Liverpool*

FOREWORD

The Linbury Trust, a grant-making charity established by Lord Sainsbury of Preston Candover, has since 1991 been the foremost supporter of UK research into chronic fatigue syndrome (CFS). The choice of this research area arose from the Trust's concern about the disabling impact of CFS on people's lives, the frequent failure to diagnose, the absence of effective patient management, the deep ignorance surrounding the condition and the lack of credible research being undertaken. A Scientific Advisory Panel was established with the remit of developing a research strategy for improving understanding of CFS and its management. The Trust saw its task as to 'prime the pump' of research, and to this end it has, to date, invested almost £4 million in a programme of science. Most of the funding went to proposals from research workers, but in areas that were judged under-served the Panel actively solicited applications — for example, CFS in childhood and adolescence, and evaluation of complementary therapies. Every part of the programme was exposed to external peer review.

The Linbury Trust and the members of the Advisory Panel wished to see CFS taken seriously, and the work done so far represents an important start. The condition is real and the patients need help. Although many of the Linbury-funded projects are still incomplete, the Panel and Trustees are sufficiently impressed by the body of evidence to make two strong recommendations: firstly, Government should acknowledge the existence and importance of CFS as a preliminary to ensuring that patients' needs are properly met; and, secondly, other funding bodies, including the National Health Service Research and Development arm and the Research Councils, should in the future offer serious support for work on the syndrome.

Seeking to record progress so far, the Trust invited Robin Fox, former editor of *The Lancet*, to make this collection of brief commentaries by present and former grant holders. The pump of CFS research is now primed and the time has come for Government and other funding bodies to carry the process forward.

Alan McGregor
Leszek Borysiewicz
Tom Craig
Richard Frackowiak
Members of the
Linbury Advisory
Panel on CFS

EDITOR'S NOTE

I picture some readers shaking their heads over this booklet. Where is dental amalgam? Where hypnotherapy or antivirals? Where organophosphates? More tellingly, why no reference to the important work of X — or why almost nothing about children? Let me explain.

The Linbury Trust gave me a free hand, and my first move was to see what had been published on chronic fatigue syndrome since the first CDC definition a decade ago. Medline offered more than 1200 references, so a panoramic view was clearly beyond the scope of the enterprise. I decided on snapshots. From the Trust's scientific programme (see Appendix) I would pick a dozen key players and invite them to write personal accounts of their special areas — what they had done, what they had learned, where we go from here. The coverage would be far from complete, in subject matter as well as references, but in just a few pages we might convey the extraordinary flowering of research on CFS. Everyone responded cheerfully to my invitations; the blame for errors of omission lies with me.

My wisest move was to enlist the aid of Dr Tony Cleare, the Linbury Trust Research Fellow, who exemplifies the critical thinking this subject needs. If some cohesion has been achieved in the booklet, much of the credit goes to him. I am especially grateful for his diagram on p. 68.

Robin Fox

EPIDEMIOLOGY

EPIDEMIOLOGY OF CFS

Simon Wessely

Epidemiology is the study of illness in populations, and epidemiologists seek to discover not only how many people suffer from a given condition but also its causes and the outcomes. Sometimes one can more easily define what epidemiology is not than what it is. Epidemiology is *not* concerned with the study of small groups of individuals seen in the hospital setting. There are many reasons for this, but the principal one is that those who attend specialist clinics do not represent the condition as it exists in nature: a large number of biases have intervened between the onset of illness and attendance at a clinic.

Chronic fatigue syndrome exemplifies the strengths of the epidemiological approach as well as the limitations of hospital-based samples. Let us start with the simplest observation — how many people suffer from CFS? Immediately we pause and ask ourselves, 'What is it?'. Until we have an agreed case definition we cannot say how much of it there is, let alone what causes it or how to treat it. Thus the beginnings of modern research on CFS can be traced to the actions of the research community during the 1980s and beyond in drawing up case definitions for the illness. Such definitions are not the last word — they can and will be changed — but they are an essential start to any research endeavour.

DEFINITIONS

The first attempt emerged from the observations of American virologists and immunologists who had noted an overlap between the symptoms of CFS and those of infectious and immunological diseases. This is known as the 1988 CDC definition, CDC being the Centers for Disease Control in Atlanta where the key meeting took place. However, this definition was rather unsatisfactory. For example, it stated that CFS was a diagnosis of exclusion, and among the things that had to be excluded were all the psychiatric conditions with which CFS might be confused. For example, if you were depressed, then you could not have CFS. This was illogical, and systematic research published shortly afterwards suggested that this process of exclusion would rule out the diagnosis of CFS in many people who were deemed by their doctors to have the illness. So a new definition was proposed, known as the 1994 CDC definition. This was more robust and, unlike the 1988 version, could be applied in the field.

Meanwhile UK researchers, of whom I was one, had convened a meeting in Oxford to produce our own definition. In the 'Oxford criteria' we insisted on mental fatigue as part of the syndrome, and put less weight on somatic symptoms. There is also an Australian definition, on similar lines.

So now we had some definitions, and could begin to address the question of how common is CFS. There had been estimates before, all of which suggested that CFS was rare — less common than multiple sclerosis, for example. However, these were all faulty, for various reasons. Some were based on observations made by clinicians working in clinics that dealt largely with CFS. Because of the numerous barriers patients must surmount before getting to these clinics, such estimates are very unsound. Others depended on asking 'key informants', usually general practitioners, how many patients with CFS they have on their books. This too is unreliable, since it depends on whether or not the GP recognizes the condition at all, and if so, what condition it is that he or she recognizes.

FATIGUE IN THE COMMUNITY

I began thinking about the epidemiological issues in 1988, having run a chronic fatigue clinic at the National Hospital for Neurology at Queen Square. This was the most specialized hospital in the country and I came to see just how limited was the information that could be gathered from that setting. Our group proposed the first large-scale epidemiological study of CFS in the UK, and it was funded by the Linbury Trust. What did we find?

In the first part of the study we surveyed over 15 000 people registered with six general practices across the south of England[1]. Because this was just a paper-and-pencil questionnaire study we were unable to study CFS *per se*, but we did obtain data on the prevalence of chronic fatigue and muscle pain. It was very common: 18% had experienced substantial fatigue for six months or longer. Fatigue, however, was 'normally' distributed — i.e. the world could not be divided into those with chronic fatigue (the ill group) and those without (the well). What we were looking at was more like blood pressure: we all have it, some have higher levels than others, and a few have such high levels that something has to be done about it, but the division between normal and high blood pressure is arbitrary.

This was the beginning of a larger study to examine the relation between common viral infections and CFS. Most of the people we had been seeing in the clinics said their illness began with a viral infection, and many felt that the infection was still in their body. However, by the time people had got to the clinic they had been ill for a long time — several years usually. At that distance in time it is impossible to sort out the sequence of events. Maybe the infection was the result, and not the cause, of illness. Maybe it was a red herring: we all have four or five such infections every year, and perhaps we only remember them if something bad happens at around the same time. So we set out to conduct a 'cohort' study, in which, instead of taking a group of people with the condition and looking back in time to find out what caused it, we take people who have just been exposed to whatever it is we think might be the cause of the illness (in this case a viral infection) and follow them up to see who develops the illness, and who does not. Hence we ended up recruiting over a thousand people who consulted their GP with a viral infection, and also another thousand people who turned up with anything other than a viral infection. It took a massive effort to follow them all up for six months to see what happened to them.

What we found was that viral infections of the kind seen commonly in primary care did not lead to any increased risk of chronic fatigue or CFS, however defined[2]. If there was a link between viral infections and CFS, either it was such a rare reaction that we missed it, or it was not associated with the common-or-garden infections that we were studying. It turns out that the latter is nearer the mark. At the same time we were conducting our study, Peter White at Bart's was doing much the same but looking specifically at glandular fever[3]; and his investigation, like ours a cohort study, provided evidence implicating glandular fever in precipitating CFS no less firm than our evidence acquitting common virus infections of the same charge. We also did a third cohort study, this time retrospective rather than prospective, looking at those who had been diagnosed with viral meningitis, often an enteroviral infection in the UK. Again, the pattern that emerged was very different from that in the main primary care study: like glandular fever, viral meningitis was associated with an increased likelihood of later CFS, although this was not a specific relationship[4]. Lately, one more infection has been added to the list of agents that can trigger CFS — Q fever[5] (unless you work in an Australian abattoir, your risk of getting this infection is low).

HOW COMMON IS CFS?

Although we had not found any evidence that common viral infections were the cause of CFS, we did find a lot of people who fulfilled the various criteria for CFS. Exactly how many depended on which criteria we used[6]. Thus, if one applied the excessively restrictive 1988 CDC criteria then the figure was 0.1%, but the more liberal 1994 criteria gave 2.6%. This seems very high, and indeed it is. That is because most of those who fulfilled the criteria were also either anxious or depressed. When interviewed they certainly did not resemble what we have come to think of as 'CFS', and sometimes it seemed more sensible, clinically, to identify their primary problem as anxiety or depression: Occam's razor (do not create more categories than you need) is a very important scientific tool. This observation raises an interesting question about operational criteria, and also about what we mean by CFS: these people fulfilled the criteria, had the right symptoms and were seriously disabled, but did not 'feel' like CFS. What do we trust — clinical judgment or standardized research? It reminds us that, when we decide whether or not to label someone as CFS, we may be subject to all sorts of biases and pressures.

Anyway, even if one excluded all of those, that still left 0.5% of primary care attenders who fulfilled criteria for CFS and nothing else. This kind of figure is now emerging from other epidemiological studies in Britain and America. In Scotland the prevalence of CFS was 0.6%, although the sample size was relatively small[7]. The Scottish researchers then did a follow-up one year later[8]. This time the prevalence of CFS was 0.7%, but they were also able to make the first estimate of the incidence of CFS, which was 370 per 100 000 (once again with wide confidence intervals, which means the true figure could be considerably lower or higher). In my opinion, 0.5% is a reasonable estimate for the prevalence of CFS in primary care[9].

One question is whether CFS, as seen in general practice, is worth worrying about. You would have to be blind not to notice the devastating impact of CFS in some of those who attend specialist clinics around the world, and various studies have attested to its economic toll on individuals, families and society. But what about the larger numbers in primary care? It would be nice to record that these people are not so impaired, but this is not so. Our primary care study showed that they too had a substantial burden of illness, and that the impact of CFS was greater in terms of personal, physical and emotional disability than that associated with angina, blood pressure, arthritis or chronic bronchitis[6].

RISK FACTORS

The prospective design of the main study meant we could make one or two more epidemiological observations about CFS. Remember that, before we recruited those coming to the surgery with a viral infection, we had screened all the population with a questionnaire that measured not only fatigue but also minor psychological symptoms. We found that indices of psychological distress (stress, depression, anxiety), recorded before an individual got the viral infection, did predict those who would go on to develop CFS[10]. We found much the same thing in viral meningitis: there was an interaction between measures of previous psychological distress, getting viral meningitis, and ending up with CFS. If you had previously suffered from depression and were then unlucky enough to get viral meningitis, you had a greatly increased chance of developing CFS[4]. This is not to say that CFS and depression are one and the same, but it does say that depression is a risk factor for CFS.

While doing the community study, we had asked people what they thought was wrong with them. This meant that we had a unique sample of people who believed they had myalgic encephalomyelitis (ME), whatever that means, but had not necessarily come forward for treatment. What could we say about them? We compared them with other people who were fatigued but who did not think their problem was ME. Those who did use the term ME to describe their condition were less psychologically distressed than the rest but more fatigued, more likely to have reduced their activities, and more disabled[11].

What other risk factors are there? A reader of the popular press around the time when ME became news could be forgiven for thinking that the main risk factor for getting the illness was coming from the middle and upper classes. Not only that, but you were particularly at risk if you belonged to certain professions, such as medicine, nursing or teaching. And the last nail in your coffin was having a particular sort of personality—hard driving, successful, conscientious to a fault, and so on. This led to the label of 'yuppie flu', which many people thought insensitive but hardly any thought untrue. Doctors, meanwhile, developed elaborate theories as to why such groups should be at special risk. Maybe those professions were more exposed to viral infections or, in an inversion of the same idea, were less exposed to viral infections as children and thus more susceptible in early adult life. Perhaps these kind of people pushed themselves too hard, and did not look after themselves properly when they got infections. Explanations of this sort are nothing new: all surfaced in accounts of the Victorian version of CFS[12]. They are also wrong.

They are wrong because of a neglect of epidemiology. (For a wider review of the epidemiological issues see Refs 9 and 13.) Observations made in specialist clinics can mislead. Thus, when we looked at the primary care population, in which 90% of those who fulfilled the criteria for CFS did not think that CFS was what was wrong with them, we found no excess of any social class or any particular profession[14]. Our clinics continue to be biased towards the successful middle classes, and that tells us a lot about how people label their own illnesses and how they gain access to specialist clinics. It does not tell us much about CFS. Epidemiology tells us that CFS is not 'yuppie flu'.

QUESTIONS AWAITING ANSWERS

Where should we be going in the future? Good research often produces more questions than answers, and epidemiology is no exception. For example, we still lack a true population study (as opposed to a primary care study). We need to know much more about the outcome of CFS: a systematic review of published studies suggested that the prognosis of CFS is poor[15], but nearly all the studies had been performed in specialist care, involving patients who had already been ill for a long time: the spectre of selection bias again raises its ugly head. Are all cases of CFS the same or are there distinct subgroups? Subgroup analysis is notoriously prone to error, but there is now the beginnings of a case for making two divisions among CFS — separation of those with acute onset from those with gradual onset[16,17]; and division of those with very long illness histories, multiple symptoms and profound disability from the larger group with shorter durations, less disability and fewer symptoms[18].

Let me close by highlighting four observations that have emerged from our work. First, CFS is by no means uncommon in primary care. Second, even in that setting it is an important cause of disability — CFS is a public health issue. Third, whereas common viral infections do not precipitate CFS, some other infections, chiefly glandular fever, do. Fourth, 'yuppie flu' is a topic for social historians and not doctors: CFS affects all classes of society.

REFERENCES

1   Pawlikowska T, Chalder T, Hirsch S, Wallace P, Wright D, Wessely S. A population based study of fatigue and psychological distress. *BMJ* 1994; **308**: 743–6

2   Wessely S, Chalder T, Hirsch S, Wallace P, Wright D. Post-infectious fatigue: a prospective study in primary care. *Lancet* 1995; **345**: 1333–8

3   White P, Grover S, Kangro H, Thomas J, Amess J, Clare A. The validity and reliability of the fatigue syndrome that follows glandular fever. *Psychol Med* 1995; **25**: 917–24

4   Hotopf M, Noah N, Wessely S. Chronic fatigue and minor psychiatric morbidity after viral meningitis: a controlled study. *J Neurol Neurosurg Psychiatry* 1996; **60**: 504–9

5   Ayres J, Flint N, Smith E, *et al*. Post-infection fatigue syndrome following Q fever. *Q J Med* 1998: 105–23

6   Wessely S, Chalder T, Hirsch S, Wallace P, Wright D. The prevalence and morbidity of chronic fatigue and chronic fatigue syndrome: a prospective primary care study. *Am J Publ Health* 1997; **87**: 1449–55

7   Lawrie S, Pelosi A. Chronic fatigue syndrome in the community: prevalence and associations. *Br J Psychiatry* 1995; **166**: 793–7

8   Lawrie S, Manders D, Geddes J, Pelosi A. A population-based incidence study of chronic fatigue. *Psychol Med* 1997; **27**: 343–53

9   Wessely S. The epidemiology of chronic fatigue syndrome. *Epidemiol Rev* 1995; **17**: 139–51

10 Wessely S, Chalder T, Hirsch S, Wallace P, Wright D. Psychological symptoms, somatic symptoms and psychiatric disorder in chronic fatigue and chronic fatigue syndrome: a prospective study in primary care. *Am J Psychiatry* 1996; **153**: 1050–9

11 Chalder T, Power M, Wessely S. Chronic fatigue in the community: "a question of attribution". *Psychol Med* 1996; **26**: 791–800

12 Wessely S, Hotopf M, Sharpe M. *Chronic Fatigue and its Syndromes*. Oxford: Oxford University Press, 1998

13 Levine P. Epidemiologic advances in chronic fatigue syndrome. *J Psychiatr Res* 1997; **31**: 7–18

14 Euba R, Chalder T, Deale A, Wessely S. A comparison of the characteristics of chronic fatigue syndrome in primary and tertiary care. *Br J Psychiatry* 1996; **168**: 121–6

15 Joyce J, Hotopf M, Wessely S. The prognosis of chronic fatigue and chronic fatigue syndrome: a systematic review. *Q J Med* 1997; **90**: 223–33

16 Mawle A, Nisenbaum R, Dobbins J, *et al*. Immune responses associated with chronic fatigue syndrome: a case–control study. *J Infect Dis* 1997; **175**: 136–41

17 DeLuca J, Johnson S, Ellis S, Natelson B. Sudden vs gradual onset of chronic fatigue syndrome differentiates individuals in cognitive and psychiatric measures. *J Psychiatr Res* 1997; **31**: 83–90

18 Hickie I, Lloyd A, Hadzi-Pavlovic D, Parker G, Bird K, Wakefield D. Can the chronic fatigue syndrome be defined by distinct clinical features? *Psychol Med* 1995; **25**: 925–35

PATHOPHYSIOLOGY

While the prevalence and severity of CFS was being elucidated as described by Simon Wessely, other groups focused on pathophysiology. Since weakness and muscle pain are prominent symptoms in CFS, a first port of call for many scientists was muscle.

MUSCLE

Malcolm J Jackson, Anne McArdle

The debilitation that characterizes chronic fatigue syndrome is crucially associated with a feeling of muscle weakness. Might this weakness be explained by some abnormality of skeletal muscle function, biochemistry or structure? This question was the starting point for extensive investigations by our group and many other researchers. Here we briefly describe our investigations and the conclusions we have drawn.

FUNCTION

In view of the emphasis CFS patients give to the complaint of muscle fatigue, we might expect careful examination to reveal functional abnormalities. Enquiring into this possibility, Edwards and co-workers found no evidence of weakness when muscles were tested either with brief stimulated contractions or with maximum voluntary contractions. However, not all patients managed to achieve the same force with maximum voluntary activation of the muscle as with stimulation; and these were judged to suffer from a reduced central 'drive' to activate the muscles[1]. There was no evidence that CFS patients became more fatigued than age and sex matched controls during cycle ergometer exercise, or that they recovered more slowly from the fatiguing exercise. Surprisingly, objective assessments of muscle function gave normal results even when the patients complained of protracted fatigue after exercise. Exercise duration was also similar in the CFS patients and controls, although the patients had higher perceived exertion scores in relation to heart rate during exercise — indicating a reduced effort sensation threshold[2].

STRUCTURE

In many muscle diseases, diagnosis depends on light or electron microscopy of muscle biopsy samples. In the past, various morphological abnormalities were reported in the muscle of patients with CFS, but the work was marred either by poor documentation or by a failure to distinguish between changes that might be due to reduced physical activity, changes that might occur in normal individuals through everyday use and changes that might reflect a primary myopathy. Our group therefore investigated a large number of patients with CFS, comparing them with patients who had myalgia alone and with healthy controls.

Samples were taken from major leg muscles (anterior tibialis or quadriceps) by needle biopsy[2]. Morphological changes were seen, but usually these affected only a small number (less than 1%) of the fibres in any biopsy specimen. These abnormalities were seen both in biopsies from CFS patients (81%) and in biopsies from controls (32%). Detailed analysis revealed no significant difference in fibre type predominance between the patients and controls and no significant differences in fibre size. Changes indicative of a minor degree of degeneration or regeneration were seen in 43% of biopsy samples from patients with CFS. Specifically we found no evidence of widespread occurrence of necrotic fibres — in contrast to published data from other workers[3].

More detailed analysis indicated that changes in glycogen content were present in occasional muscle fibres from 22% of patients. These changes are assumed to reflect differences in the functional activity of a minority of fibres. Ultrastructural examination of muscle biopsies was also undertaken to look for evidence of degenerative changes and specifically to explore the possibility that CFS muscle would show mitochondrial abnormalities. A very low frequency of mitochondrial abnormalities was seen — again contrary to the suggestions of others[4]. Most importantly in this area, a retrospective comparison revealed no relation between the prevalence of morphological abnormalities and the symptom pattern in patients with CFS and/or myalgia[2].

BIOCHEMISTRY

Several groups have compared the RNA content of muscle samples from CFS patients and controls and all have observed a clear reduction[1,5,6]. These data suggest that muscle from patients with CFS has a lesser capacity to synthesize protein. To determine whether such changes have any functional significance, *in-vivo* rates of whole-body protein synthesis and quadriceps muscle protein synthesis were assessed by measurement of [^{13}C]-leucine incorporation[7]. Reductions in both muscle protein synthesis rate and whole-body protein synthesis rate were observed. The fact that such changes are present in the absence of any major abnormalities of lean body mass or muscle protein content[5,6] indicates that compensatory changes (reductions) in the rate of muscle protein degradation must have occurred to maintain muscle protein content and muscle bulk. So what do they mean? In our view, they are more likely to reflect a secondary consequence of a general reduction in habitual activity in CFS patients than to indicate an underlying muscle disorder[6].

BIOENERGETICS

When case reports suggested that individual CFS patients might have abnormalities in energy production, various approaches were applied to the study of energy metabolism in muscle. Edwards and co-workers[1] have argued that the most powerful evidence against any defect in muscle energy supply, as a cause of CFS, is that the symptoms are present at rest, before any exercise is undertaken. This contrasts strongly with the exercise-related myalgia and fatigue of patients with genetically determined biochemical defects that impair energy supply to muscle.

There is no clear evidence of abnormal muscle glycolysis in CFS, but some workers have claimed either a specific reduction or a general reduction in oxidative capacity[1,4]. Looking at mitochondrial enzyme activity, our group observed a non-specific reduction[1]. Arnold and co-workers[8], using *in-vivo* [31]P nuclear magnetic resonance techniques, initially reported that one patient with CFS had an abnormal tendency to develop intracellular acidosis with moderate aerobic exercise. In a subsequent study these investigators confirmed the presence of such changes in a small proportion of patients but could find no consistent abnormalities of glycolysis, mitochondrial metabolism or pH regulation in a group of 46 CFS patients as a whole[9]. They concluded that their data did not support the hypothesis that any specific metabolic abnormality underlies fatigue in CFS. Our group likewise found a general reduction in the activity of mitochondrial enzymes in patients with CFS and looked for evidence that enzymes coded on the mitochondrial genome might be differentially affected, compared with those coded on the nuclear genome. No such evidence was found[6].

VIRAL INFECTION

Perhaps the most contentious issue relating to muscle in CFS patients is whether there is evidence for a persistent virus infection. Patients frequently report that the illness began after a virus infection[10] and numerous viruses have been implicated, including herpesviruses, retroviruses and enteroviruses. Although there is considerable support for this idea[11–16], by no means all the evidence is positive[17–20]. Enteroviruses have attracted particular interest (see p. 14), and in our study we used essentially the same techniques by which Gow *et al.*[21,22] obtained evidence of enteroviral infection in muscle from CFS patients. We found no evidence of such infection; nor could we reproduce their data indicating that a variable proportion of samples from the control group contained enterovirus sequences. A possible explanation for these discrepant results is that the study populations of CFS patients were different. The proportion of patients reporting an acute onset of CFS after a fever was 100% in Gow's group but only 58% in ours. In the patients studied by our group we have no direct evidence that persistent viral infection plays any role in the progression of CFS, and the matter remains deeply controversial.

CONCLUSIONS

Despite extensive investigations we have no clear evidence that CFS is a muscle disorder. Many of the reported changes within CFS muscle can be attributed to a reduction in habitual activity. Additionally, we find no evidence of persistent enterovirus infection in muscle of our patients, although we cannot exclude the possibility that viral infection occurs in the initial stages of the disease.

Our group has hypothesized that a vicious circle of biochemical changes arises in CFS, consequent upon various initial insults that might include mental depression or debilitating viral infection. This initial insult leads to inactivity, with ensuing reduction in muscle mitochondrial enzyme activities. This would result in exercise intolerance, muscle pain in exercise and hence further inactivity on exercise[23]. Such a hypothesis reconciles many of the apparently contradictory and confusing data from studies of muscle in CFS and provides a framework for further studies and therapeutic strategies.

ACKNOWLEDGEMENTS

We acknowledge the contributions of many former co-workers, particularly Professor Richard Edwards, Dr Anton Wagenmakers and Dr Peter MacLennan.

REFERENCES

1   Edwards RHT, Newham DJ, Peters TJ. Muscle biochemistry and pathophysiology in postviral fatigue syndrome. *Br Med Bull* 1991; **47**: 826–37

2   Edwards RHT, Gibson H, Clague JE, Helliwell TR. Muscle histopathology and physiology in the chronic fatigue syndrome. In: Bock GR, Whelan J. eds. *Chronic Fatigue Syndrome*. Chichester: Wiley, 1993: 102–31

3   Behan PO, Behan WHM, Bell EJ. The postviral fatigue syndrome — analysis of the findings in 50 cases. *J Infect* 1985; **10**: 211–22

4   Behan WHM. Muscles, mitochondria and myalgia. *J Pathol* 1992; **166**: 213–14

5   Preedy VR, Smith DG, Salisbury JR, Peters TJ. Biochemical and muscle studies in patients with acute onset post-viral fatigue syndrome. *J Clin Pathol* 1993; **46**: 722–6

6   McArdle A, McArdle F, Jackson MJ, Page SF, Fahal I, Edwards RHT. Investigation by polymerase chain reaction of enteroviral infection in patients with chronic fatigue syndrome. *Clin Sci* 1996; **90**: 295–300

7   Pacy PJ, Read M, Peters TJ, Halliday D. Post-absorptive whole body leucine kinetics and quadriceps muscle protein synthetic rate in the post-viral syndrome. *Clin Sci* 1988; **75**: 36–7P

8   Arnold DL, Bore PJ, Radda GK. Excessive intracellular acidosis of skeletal muscle on exercise in a patient with a post-viral exhaustion/fatigue syndrome. *Lancet* 1984; **i**: 1367–9

9   Barnes RJ, Taylor DJ, Kemp GJ, Radda GK. Skeletal muscle bioenergetics in the chronic fatigue syndrome. *J Neurol Neurosurg Psychiatry* 1993; **56**: 679–83

10 Fekety R. Infection and chronic fatigue syndrome. In: Straus SE, ed. *Chronic Fatigue Syndrome*. New York: Marcel Dekker, 1994: 101–80

11 Buchwald D, Cheney PR, Peterson DL, *et al.* A chronic illness characterized by fatigue, neurologic and immunologic disorders, and active human herpesvirus type 6 infection. *Ann Intern Med* 1992; **116**: 103–13

12 Holmes GP, Kaplan JE, Stewart JA, *et al.* A cluster of patients with a chronic mononucleosis-like syndrome. Is Epstein–Barr virus the cause? *JAMA* 1987; **257**: 2297–302

13 Natelson BH, Ye N, Moul DE, *et al.* High titres of Epstein–Barr virus DNA polymerase are found in patients with severe fatiguing illness. *J Med Virol* 1994; **42**: 42–6

14 DeFreitas E, Hilliard B, Cheney PR, *et al.* Retroviral sequences related to human 5666 T-lymphotropic virus type II in patients with chronic fatigue immune dysfunction syndrome. *Proc Natn Acad Sci USA* 1991; **81**: 2922–6

15 Archard LC, Bowles NE, Behan PO, *et al.* Post-viral fatigue syndrome: persistence of enterovirus RNA in muscle and elevated creatine kinase. *J R Soc Med* 1988; **81**: 326–9

16 Bowles NE, Bayston TA, Zhang H, *et al.* Persistence of enterovirus RNA in muscle biopsy samples. *J Med* 1993; **24**: 145–60

17 Straus SE. Studies of herpes virus infection in chronic fatigue syndrome. In: Bock GR, Whelan J, eds. *Chronic Fatigue Syndrome*. Chichester: Wiley, 1993: 132–59

18 Folks TM, Heneine W, Khan AS, *et al.* Investigation of retroviral involvement in chronic fatigue syndrome. In: Bock GR, Whelan J, eds. *Chronic Fatigue Syndrome*. Chichester: Wiley, 1993: 160–75

19 Khan AS, Heneine WM, Chapman LE, *et al.* Assessment of retrovirus sequence and possible risk factors for the involvement in chronic fatigue syndrome in adults. *Ann Intern Med* 1993; **118**: 241–5

20 Heneine W, Woods TC, Sinha SD, *et al.* Lack of evidence for infection with known human and animal retroviruses in patients with chronic fatigue syndrome. *Clin Infect Dis* 1994; **18** (suppl 1): S121–5

21 Gow JW, Behan WHM, Clements GB, Woodall C, Riding M, Behan PO. Enteroviral RNA sequences detected by polymerase chain reaction in muscle of patients with postviral fatigue syndrome. *BMJ* 1991; **302**: 692–6

22 Gow JW, Behan WHM, Simpson K, *et al.* Studies on enterovirus in patients with chronic fatigue syndrome. *Clin Infect Dis* 1994; **18** (suppl 1): S126–9

23 Wagenmakers AJM, Kaur N, Coakley J, *et al.* Mitochondrial metabolism in myopathy and myalgia. In: Benzi G, ed. *Advances in Myochemistry*. London: John Libbey Eurotext, 1987: 219–30

Although abnormalities in muscle have been found, CFS is clearly not a primary muscle disorder. Many of the observed changes might be secondary to the effects of illness. Another characteristic feature perceived by patients is the onset after an infection of some sort. Malcolm Jackson and Anne McArdle found no evidence of persistent viral infection in their patients; however, at the same time Dr Clements and co-workers were funded to pursue the notion that a specific viral infection might underlie CFS.

ENTEROVIRUSES

G B Clements

Ever since the Iceland and Royal Free outbreaks, there has been much speculation regarding the possible involvement of viruses in pathogenesis of chronic fatigue syndrome. Particularly favoured candidates have been Epstein–Barr virus, cytomegalovirus, human herpesvirus 6 and enteroviruses. Our group has focused on enteroviruses.

So named because of their association with the alimentary tract, enteroviruses form a genus of the Picornaviridae family and are small non-enveloped RNA viruses. The best known members are the three types of poliovirus but others include Echo and Coxsackie viruses. Poliomyelitis apart, enteroviruses have been implicated in such disorders as aseptic meningitis, myocarditis, hepatitis and encephalitis.

Initially, the laboratory evidence for an association between enterovirus infection and CFS was serological: antibodies to enteroviruses were detected more frequently and at a higher level in CFS patients than in controls[1-3]. CFS might simply be triggered by acute enteroviral infection, with some other mechanism supervening, or it might be maintained by persistent infection. Enterovirus persistence has been demonstrated in children with agammaglobulinaemia[4] and in some cases of cardiomyopathy. Our research concentrates on the identification and characterization of atypical enteroviral sequences observed in some CFS patients in the West of Scotland and elsewhere. In muscle biopsy specimens, such sequences have been detected more frequently in CFS patients than in controls[5,6].

EVIDENCE FOR ENTEROVIRUS INFECTION IN CFS

We have used the sensitive polymerase chain reaction (PCR) to amplify and detect a region of the enterovirus genome in patients presenting with CFS. The first-round primers are designed to amplify a 414-nucleotide fragment of the highly conserved 5′ non-translated region (NTR) of the enterovirus sequence, and then second-round primers amplify an internal 264-nucleotide region. Where possible, amplification is followed by direct nucleic acid sequencing and comparison with several documented enterovirus sequences.

We screened the serum of 88 chronic fatigue patients from whom samples had been taken during 1990–1991[7]. In addition, buffy coat specimens and stool specimens from some patients were examined. Samples from two cohorts of comparison individuals were obtained — first, acutely ill individuals with symptoms consistent with enteroviral infection (matched by age, sex, and date of receipt of specimen); and, second, healthy individuals matched by age and date of receipt of specimen. Before onset of fatigue more than half the CFS patients had had an influenza-like respiratory illness. Enterovirus-specific sequences were detected in 36 of 88 serum samples from chronic fatigue patients, 22 of 82 acutely ill individuals, and 3 of 126 healthy individuals (Table 1). The enteroviral PCR positivity did not correlate with any particular features of chronic fatigue such as myalgia or sleep disturbance or depression, nor did it reflect any history of illness at onset of fatigue (Table 2). These results add to the evidence for persistent enterovirus infection in a proportion of CFS patients. But what sort of enteroviruses? Galbraith et al.[8] compared the nucleotide sequences of the 5′-NTR PCR products with known enteroviral sequences and found them to be atypical. They used phylogenetic analysis to compare sequences associated with CFS and those from enteroviruses causing acute infections. The inferred phylogenetic tree identified three groupings, one of which correlated with the diagnosis of CFS (Figure 1). Indicating a

Table 1. *Results of second-round PCR on specimens from chronic fatigue (CF) patients and comparison groups*

Specimen	Number	Positive	Negative
CF serum	88	36	52
Comparison A serum	82	22	60
Comparison B serum	126	3	123
CF stool	31	15	16
Comparison A stool	32	9	23
CF buffy coat	62	17	45
Total	421	102	319

Table 2. *Enteroviral polymerase chain reaction (PCR) results from chronic fatigue patients and history of illness at onset of fatigue*

	Enterovirus PCR positive	Enterovirus PCR negative
No previous illness	1	7
Respiratory infection	21	27
Gastrointestinal upset	3	5
Myalgia	2	4
Sore throat	6	6
Other infections	11	13
No history given	6	6
Total	50	68

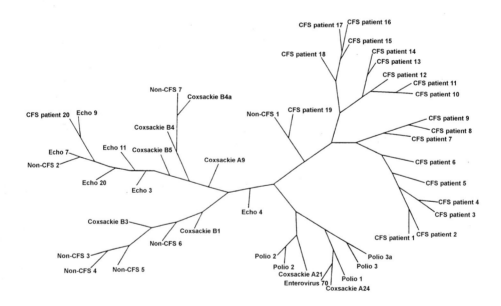

Figure 1

Phylogenetic tree (from Ref 8).

close relationship between the CFS enteroviral sequences the analysis showed that 19 of 20 were distinct from previously described enteroviruses. The fact that no correlation was found between the results of Coxsackie B1-5 neutralization tests and the 5'-NTR enterovirus PCR status of sera[9] offered further evidence that this was a novel group of enteroviruses, possibly of causal relevance in some cases of CFS.

We elected to follow CFS patients prospectively, correlating clinical symptoms with the presence or absence of enteroviral sequences. A questionnaire was developed in cooperation with the clinicians of Ruchill Hospital to monitor the pattern of symptoms in CFS cases. Patients have been recalled every twelve months to complete a repeat questionnaire and to provide a further blood sample for PCR analysis. Preliminary data have shown persistence of enteroviral sequences in a proportion of patients[10]. 8 of the 106 individuals were positive for enteroviral sequences, detected by PCR in two serum samples taken at least five months apart; and in 4 of these individuals the nucleotide sequence of the 5'-NTR (bases 174–423) was virtually identical in the two samples. The sequence pairs also each had a unique shared pattern indicating that the virus had persisted. In one further individual there had clearly been infection with two different enteroviruses. In the remaining 3, the lack of unique shared features suggested recurrent rather than persistent infection.

Collaboration with the group at Cardiff has provided data on responses to polio vaccination[11]. The effects of live oral poliovirus vaccination were examined, double-blind, in CFS patients and controls. CFS patients were allocated randomly to placebo ($n=7$) or vaccine ($n=7$); all controls received the vaccine. Vaccine administration did not exacerbate CFS, but the laboratory results of patients differed distinctly from those of controls— increased poliovirus isolation; earlier peak proliferative responses; lower T-cell subsets on certain days post-vaccination; and a trend for less gamma-interferon. Thus, although the investigators concluded that polio vaccination can safely be performed in CFS, the study yielded evidence of altered immune reactivity and virus clearance.

WORK IN PROGRESS

In future we shall determine nucleotide sequences in additional genomic regions and/or the entire genome of the atypical enteroviruses present in certain CFS patients. Subsequent sequence analyses and comparison with the known enteroviral sequences will define the classification of the associated enteroviruses. The question of persistence will be further explored by longitudinal follow-up of patients throughout their illness and comparison of enteroviral sequences obtained from given individuals. Within the limits of detection of the existing 5'-NTR PCR, this will define whether the enterovirus associated with CFS persists for long periods in affected patients. In work soon to be published we have followed a cohort of CFS patients and related the enterovirus results to clinical course, as revealed by answers to a questionnaire.

REFERENCES

1 Fegan KG, Behan PO, Bell EJ. Myalgic encephalomyelitis — report of an epidemic. *J R Coll Gen Practit* 1983; **33**: 335–7

2 Bell EJ, McCartney RA. A study of Coxsackie B virus infections 1972–1983. *J Hyg* 1984; **93**: 197–203

3 Bell EJ, McCartney R, Riding MH. Coxsackie B viruses and myalgic encephalomyelitis. *J R Soc Med* 1988; **81**: 329–31

4 O'Neill KM, Pallansch MA, Winkelstein JA, *et al*. Chronic group A coxsackievirus infection in agammaglobulinemia: demonstration of genomic variation of serotypically identical isolates persistently excreted by the same patients. *J Infect Dis* 1988; **157**: 183–6

5 Archard LC, Bowles NE, Behan PO, *et al*. Postviral fatigue syndrome: persistence of enterovirus RNA in muscle and elevated creatine kinase. *J R Soc Med* 1988; **81**: 326–9

6 Gow JW, Behan WMH, Clements GB, Woodall C, Riding M, Behan PO. Enteroviral RNA sequences detected by polymerase chain reaction in muscle of patients with postviral fatigue syndrome. *BMJ* 1991; **302**: 692–6

7 Clements GB, McGarry F, Nairn C, Galbraith DN. Detection of enterovirus-specific RNA in serum: the relationship to chronic fatigue. *J Med Virol* 1995; **45**: 156–61

8 Galbraith DN, Nairn C, Clements GB. Phylogenetic analysis of short enteroviral sequences from patients with chronic fatigue syndrome. *J Gen Virol* 1995; **76**: 1701–7

9 Nairn C, Clements GB, Galbraith DN. Comparison of coxsackie B neutralisation and enteroviral PCR in chronic fatigue patients. *J Med Virol* 1995; **46**(4): 310–13

10 Galbraith DN, Nairn C, Clements GB. Evidence for enteroviral persistence in humans. *J Gen Virol* 1997; **78**: 307–12

11 Vedhara K, Llewelyn MB, Fox JD, Jones M, Jones R, Clements GB, Wang ECY, Smith AP, Borysiewicz LK. Consequences of live poliovirus vaccine administration in chronic fatigue syndrome. *J Neuroimmunol* 1997; **75**: 183–95

Any link to an acute or chronic infection needs to take account of the patient's immune status. Many patients not only claim that their CFS started after an infection; they also believe they get viral infections more frequently and more severely during the illness

DISTURBED IMMUNITY

Phillip Cash, Beatriz Gimenez

Many researchers, over the years, have tried to explain the diverse features of chronic fatigue syndrome in terms of disturbed immunity. For example, persistent infections and their associated chronic symptoms may develop through an inadequate immune response. In addition, abnormal cytokine levels, interacting with the central nervous system, could cause fever, myalgia and sleep disturbance. Some researchers have also sought immunological markers that might allow objective laboratory diagnosis of the condition. Interest in the immune status of CFS patients was originally stimulated by suggestions that the onset of CFS was preceded by an infection. In the case of virus infection the notion of chronic infection was mooted, with disturbed immunity either the cause or the effect. Lately, the picture has been complicated by evidence of malfunction in the hypothalamus-pituitary axis (HPA). This might be related to disturbed immunity because the HPA and immune system seem to interact; for example, interleukin 1 and interleukin 6 can influence the HPA, and neuropeptides released by the anterior pituitary can influence the immune system[1]. In these studies interpretation is made difficult by variation between laboratories: this is partly due to differences in technique, but more fundamentally arises from heterogeneity in the populations. Here we discuss some of the immunological indices that have been commonly examined in CFS patients.

CELL-MEDIATED IMMUNITY

Cell-mediated immune responses are the function of specific lymphocyte populations, differentiated in the laboratory by the expression of CD molecules on the cell surface. CD markers are detected by use of specific antibodies, and the cells expressing them are quantified in a fluorescence-activated cell sorter. In an early study, Lloyd et al.[2] found lower absolute numbers of circulating helper (CD4+) and cytotoxic (CD8+) T cells than in controls but these results were not confirmed by later investigators using healthy controls matched for age and sex[3,4]. As regards the proportions of CD4+ and CD8+ T cells, no consistent differences have been found between CFS patients and healthy individuals[5,6].

One of the strongest findings from analysis of lymphocyte populations in CFS relates to natural killer (NK) cells — which are part of the innate immune system that acts against tumour cells and virus-infected cells. Two groups[6,7] report that, compared with healthy subjects, circulating NK cells from CFS patients had a low level of cytotoxicity under standard assay conditions. Regarding numbers or percentages of NK cells, both decreases[8,9] and increases[10] have been reported. Improvement in the quality of life for CFS patients with low NK cell activity has been reported following administration of interferon-α[11], which is known to boost the activity of NK cells.

CYTOKINES

Cytokines act as intercellular messengers, regulating the cells comprising the immune system. Differences between CFS patients and healthy controls in the levels of circulating cytokines and, in some instances, their corresponding soluble receptors have been the focus of several investigations[8]. Linde[12] and Patarca[13] and co-workers reported raised interleukin-1α (IL-1α) in CFS serum, and Lloyd *et al.*[14] found raised interferon-α in cerebrospinal fluid. At least in the case of IL-1α the abnormality was not specific for CFS since similar results were obtained in infectious mononucleosis[12]. Bennett and co-workers[15] reported that transforming growth factor β levels in CSF patients were higher not only than those in healthy controls but also than those in patients with fatigue of other origins ('disease controls'). However, other workers did not find significant differences in TGF-β expression[16]. One reason for such discordant results may be that data on cytokine expression vary between laboratories.

IN-VITRO ASSAYS

T-cell proliferation after exposure to phytohaemagglutinin (PHA) is a common marker for T-cell function. In general, CFS patients show lower levels of PHA stimulated proliferation than healthy subjects[6]; and, under similar conditions of PHA stimulation, IL-2 expression by T cells is also less[17]. The latter observation contrasts with the serum levels of IL-2, which are higher in CFS patients than in healthy individuals[18]. Recently, the activities of the immune cells have been determined in the absence of external stimuli — a good way to examine immune status since it reflects more closely the *in-vivo* state of the cells. In the absence of stimuli, T cell proliferation is higher for CFS patients[19], and the ability to distinguish between CFS patients and healthy subjects was improved when cytokine expression was determined in unstimulated cell cultures[20]. We made a similar observation for IL-1β expression by unstimulated monocytes grown *in vitro* (unpublished).

The capacity of monocytes to express cytokines and other markers of function has been studied in CFS patients. Two research groups[9,21] found, in most CFS patients, subnormal phagocytic indices as well as decreased expression of HLA-DR antigens and Fc and C3b receptors, but increased expression of intracellular adhesion molecule 1 and lymphocyte function associated antigen 1. Barker *et al.*[22], however, reported that neither monocyte phagocytosis nor the production of superoxide anion distinguished CFS patients from healthy controls. Data from our laboratory (unpublished) indicate that monocytes from most CFS patients show abnormal *in-vitro* maturation.

HUMORAL IMMUNITY

The humoral arm of the immune system comprises the antibody response arising from B-cell activation. Imbalances in the subclasses of immunoglobulins have been described in CFS. For example, Lloyd *et al.*[2] reported depression in the IgG1 and IgG3 subclasses, though this observation was not confirmed by others[9]. Naturally, many groups have looked at antibodies in relation to infection hypotheses but we shall not discuss this work here. What about autoimmunity? Autoantibodies have been found against nuclear antigens[23], with at least some of the response directed towards the cellular proteins lamin B and vimentin[24,25], serotonin, gangliosides and phospholipids[26].

CONCLUSIONS AND FUTURE STUDIES

Many of the results in CFS patients are consistent with chronic low-level activation of the immune system together with depressed cell-mediated immunity (reflected, for example, by low NK cell activity). The cause of the disturbance remains unknown. Indeed, we do not know whether it is primary or secondary: are certain individuals at risk because of a pre-existing abnormality in their immune system, developing the syndrome because of some secondary event; or is the immune dysfunction a response to some as yet unknown primary cause? In the case of a viral cause of CFS, one can readily understand how an existing defect might hamper clearance and allow progression to chronic infection. Alternatively, both Epstein–Barr virus and Coxsackie B virus, among the apparent initiators of CFS, are capable of infecting cells in the immune system[27,28] and disturbing immunity in that way.

On many issues the data are hard to interpret. What is the way forward? One important question is whether immune status is related to severity of the illness. Looking at lymphocyte subsets, Peakman[10] found no such relation; but Hassan[19] and Landay[4] found that severity scores were related, respectively, to HLA expression on CD4+ cells and the levels of CD8+ and CD38+ T-cells. Future studies must go beyond the analysis of lymphocyte subsets and include measurements of cytokine expression and monocyte function.

The quest for an immunological marker of CFS has so far been unavailing. We have referred to the difficulties of laboratory standardization, but a more important obstacle may be patient heterogeneity[29]. When immunological abnormalities are detected, they tend to be found in some CFS patients but not all. A final answer to the immunological enigmas of CFS will depend on strict standardization of assay systems and rigorous definition of patient populations.

REFERENCES

1   Goetzl EJ, Sreedharan SP. Mediators of communication and adaptation in the neuroendocrine and immune system. *FASEB J* 1992; **6**: 2646–52

2   Lloyd AR, Wakefield D, Boughton CR, Dwyer JM. Immunological abnormalities in the chronic fatigue syndrome. *Med J Aust* 1989; **151**: 122–4

3   Tirelli U, Bernardi D, Importa S, Pinto A. Immunologic abnormalities in chronic fatigue syndrome. *Scand J Immunol* 1994; **40**: 601–8

4   Landay AL, Jessop C, Lennette ET, Levy JA. Chronic fatigue syndrome: clinical condition associated with immune activation. *Lancet* 1991; **338**: 707–12

5   Buchwald D, Cheney PR, Peterson DL, *et al.* A chronic illness characterized by fatigue, neurologic and immunologic disorders, and active human herpesvirus type 6 infection. *Ann Intern Med* 1992; **116**: 103–13

6   Klimas NG, Salvato FR, Morgan R, Fletcher MA. Immunologic abnormalities in chronic fatigue syndrome. *J Clin Microbiol* 1990; **28**: 1403–10

7   Ojo-Amaize EA, Conley EJ, Peter JB. Decreased natural killer cell activity is associated with severity of chronic fatigue immune dysfunction syndrome. *Clin Infect Dis* 18 (suppl 1): S157–9

8   Tirelli U, Bernardi D, Importa S, Pinto A. Immunologic abnormalities in chronic fatigue syndrome. *J Chron Fatigue Synd* 1994; **2**: 85–96

9   Gupta S, Vayuvegula B. A comprehensive immunological analysis in chronic fatigue syndrome. *Scand J Immunol* 1991; **33**: 319–27

10   Peakman M, Deale A, Field R, Mahalingam M, Wessely S. Clinical improvement in chronic fatigue syndrome is not associated with lymphocyte subsets of function or activation. *Clin Immunopathol* 1997; **82**: 83–91

11   See DM, Tilles JG. Alpha-interferon treatment of patients with chronic fatigue syndrome. *Immunol Invest* 1996; **25**: 153–64

12   Linde A, Andersson B, Svenson SB, *et al.* Serum levels of lymphokines and soluble cellular receptors in primary Epstein–Barr virus infection and in patients with chronic fatigue syndrome. *J Infect Dis* 1992; **165**: 994–1000

13   Patarca R, Limas NG, Lugtendorf S, *et al.* Dysregulated expression of tumor necrosis factor in chronic fatigue syndrome: interrelations with cellular sources and patterns of soluble immune mediator expression. *Clin Infect Dis* 18 (suppl 1): S147–53

14   Lloyd AR, Hickie I, Brockman A, *et al.* Serum and cerebrospinal fluid cytokine levels in patients with chronic fatigue syndrome and control subjects. *J Infect Dis* 1991; **164**: 1023–4

15   Bennett AL, Chao CC, Hu S, *et al.* Elevation of bioactive transforming growth factor-beta in serum from patients with chronic fatigue syndrome. *J Clin Immunol* 1997; **17**: 160–6

16   Swanink CM, Vercoulen JH, Galama JM, *et al.*
      Lymphocyte subsets, apoptosis, and cytokines in
      patients with chronic fatigue syndrome. *J Infect
      Dis* 1996; **173**: 460–3

17   Gold D, Bowden R, Sixbey J, *et al.* Chronic
      fatigue. A prospective clinical and virologic study.
      JAMA 1990; **264**: 48–53

18   Cheney PR, Dorman SE, Bell DS. Interleukin-2
      and the chronic fatigue syndrome. *Ann Intern Med*
      1989; **110**: 321

19   Hassan IS, Bannister BA, Akbar A, *et al.* A study of
      the immunology of the chronic fatigue syndrome:
      correlation of immunologic parameters to health
      dysfunction. *Clin Immunol Immunopathol* (in press)

20   Gupta S, Aggarwal S, See D, Starr A. Cytokine
      production by adherent and non-adherent mono-
      nuclear cells in chronic fatigue syndrome. *J
      Psychiatr Res* 1997; **31**: 149–56

21   Prieto J, Subira ML, Castilla A, Serrano M.
      Naloxone-reversible monocyte dysfunction in
      patients with chronic fatigue syndrome. *Scand J
      Immunol* 1989; **30**: 13–20

22   Barker E, Fujimura SF, Fadem MB, *et al.*
      Immunologic abnormalities associated with
      chronic fatigue syndrome. *Clin Infect Dis* 1994;
      18 (suppl 1): S136–41

23   Bates DW, Buchwald D, Lee J, *et al.* Clinical
      laboratory findings in patients with chronic
      fatigue syndrome. *Arch Intern Med* 1995; **155**:
      97–103

24   Konstantinov K, von Mikecz A, Buchwald D, *et al.*
      Autoantibodies to nuclear envelope antigens in
      chronic fatigue syndrome. *J Clin Invest* 1996; **98**:
      1888–96

25   von Mikecz A, Konstantinov K, Buchwald DS, *et
      al.* High frequency of autoantibodies to insoluble
      cellular antigens in patients with chronic fatigue
      syndrome. *Arthritis Rheum* 1997; **40**: 295–305

26   Klein R, Berg PA. High incidence of antibodies to
      5-hydroxytryptamine, gangliosides and phospho-
      lipids in patients with chronic fatigue and
      fibromyalgia syndrome and their relatives: evi-
      dence for a clinical entity of both disorders. *Eur J
      Med Res* 1995; **1**: 21–6

27   Jones JF. Serologic and immunologic responses in
      chronic fatigue syndrome with emphasis on the
      Epstein–Barr virus. *Rev Infect Dis* 1991; **13** (suppl
      1): S26–31

28   Gimenez HB, Amarasekera DS, Argo E, Cash P.
      Analysis of protein synthesis by 2-dimensional gel
      electrophoresis in T cells persistently infected with
      coxsackie B virus. *Electrophoresis* 1995; **16**: 317–21

29   Mawle AC, Nisenbaum R, Dobbins JG, *et al.*
      Immune responses associated with chronic fatigue
      syndrome: a case–control study. *J Infect Dis* 1997;
      175: 136–41

Many researchers speculated that the primary dysfunction underlying CFS was at some level in the brain. An early observation was that CFS was associated with a higher rate of psychological disturbances than might have been expected. Trudie Chalder describes the findings in this area, and a way to integrate the psychological disturbances with the syndrome as a whole.

BRAIN

Psychosocial aspects

Trudie Chalder

Why is chronic fatigue syndrome such a contentious issue? At the heart of the debate is an outmoded dualistic notion of illness whereby the mind and body are assumed to operate separately. Thus, CFS the physical disease is seen as legitimate, CFS the psychological illness as malingering.

A MULTIFACTORIAL MODEL

Because of the subjective heterogeneous nature of the condition, it seems that a complex interaction of physiological, cognitive, behavioural and affective components is responsible for both its development and its maintenance. A cognitive behavioural model, proposed by our group ten years ago, takes into account such factors[1]. The model suggests that, while life stress and infections may contribute to the onset of fatigue, several different factors such as avoidance of activity may be contributing to its perpetuation.

There are good reasons for developing such theoretical models. Clearly, one hopes that better understanding will lead to effective treatments; and in the case of CFS this is just what happened. Two randomized controlled trials have clearly demonstrated the benefits of cognitive behavioural therapy[2,3] (see p. 59).

Randomized controlled trials not only contribute to our knowledge about treatment but also add to our understanding of the condition. However, in people with longstanding illnesses it is impossible to be sure what contributed to the onset. With funding from the Linbury Trust we conducted a series of studies in primary care as part of a longitudinal prospective examination of the role of viruses in determining chronic fatigue. The common aim was to investigate factors that were hypothesized to be contributing to both its development and its perpetuation. Our clinical experience had suggested that, while viral infection might be a necessary trigger of the symptom, it was unlikely to be a sufficient explanation for symptom chronicity. Rather, an interaction of factors would be implicated.

Study 1

The aim of the first study was to determine the prevalence of fatigue and its association with psychological distress in the general population. Fatigue and psychological distress were correlated and were continuously distributed. Although the two constructs overlap the correlation is not a perfect one, so there may be differences in terms of factors which predict the development of the disorder[4].

Study 2

In the second study we looked at the roles of life events, social support and lack of fitness or poor physical condition (as indicated by reported breathlessness on exertion), in the development of fatigue in primary care. Negative life events, perceived lack of emotional support and lack of fitness were associated with the onset of fatigue and with its severity once established. Perceived lack of practical support and lack of fitness were specific associations of chronic fatigue[5].

Study 3

In the third study we examined the roles of life events, social support and coping in the maintenance of fatigue. Negative life events and lack of social support were independent associations of chronicity of fatigue. The association between life events and chronicity of fatigue was stronger when levels of reported social support were high (interaction effect). This is the reverse of what one sees in depression, where social support buffers the effect of life events[6]. Cognitive coping — i.e. trying to see the positive side of the situation — was negatively associated with chronicity, so this may act as a protective factor[5].

Study 4

The fourth study followed up three samples of fatigued subjects in the community according to whether they attributed their symptom to 'ME' (myalgic encephalomyelitis), psychological problems or social problems. ME attributers had the lowest scores of depression/anxiety but the worst social adjustment. Of the three, 'social' attributers were least socially impaired, while their depression and anxiety scores were intermediate between those with ME and psychological attributions. Depression and anxiety were highest in the group with psychological attributions[7]. In terms of coping, a reduction of activity as a way of coping with fatigue was associated with greater disability. There is some preliminary evidence that patients with CFS reduce activity in response to cognitions related to the fear of making symptoms worse[8].

Study 5

In this final study we evaluated the efficacy of a self-help booklet and specific advice in reducing fatigue in a group of individuals with chronic fatigue. A self-help intervention was compared with no treatment. Both groups improved, but the self-help group achieved a better outcome[9].

These studies support the idea that fatigue is best understood within the context of a complex multifactorial model that distinguishes between predisposing, precipitating and perpetuating factors.

FUTURE DIRECTIONS

Future research should be directed towards clarifying the predisposing, precipitating and perpetuating factors in fatigue states. To date, very little research has been done on predisposing factors, probably because of cost and time. Longitudinal epidemiological research, although informative, is very difficult. However, in order to ascertain more about childhood factors and their influence on development, such investigations are essential. We need to learn much more about the relative contributions of and interactions between personality, coping and early life experiences.

The role of social support and life events in precipitating fatigue need futher investigation—in particular, the inverse buffering effect.

Factors that maintain fatigue once it has been triggered also need further attention. There is already some evidence that illness beliefs and coping interact to maintain both fatigue and disability[10,11], but the influence of personality has been somewhat neglected. Although there may be some truth in the stereotype of the CFS patient as being conscientious and successful, with high personal standards[12,13], the more conventional means of measuring personality constructs, such as extraversion and introversion, could be more revealing.

REFERENCES

1   Butler S, Chalder T, Ron M, Wessely S. Cognitive behaviour therapy in chronic fatigue syndrome. *J Neurol Neurosurg Psychiatry* 1991; **54**: 153–8

2   Sharpe M, Hawton K, Simkin S, *et al.* Cognitive behaviour therapy for the chronic fatigue syndrome: a randomized controlled trial. *BMJ* 1996; **312**: 22–6

3   Deale A, Chalder T, Marks I, Wessely S. A randomised controlled trial of cognitive behaviour versus relaxation therapy for chronic fatigue syndrome. *Am J Psychiatry* 1997; **154**: 408–14

4   Pawlikowska T, Chalder T, Hirsch S, Wallace P, Wright D, Wessely S. A population based study of fatigue and psychological distress. *BMJ* 1994; **308**: 743–6

5   Chalder T. *Factors Contributing to the Development and Maintenance of Fatigue.* PhD thesis, University of London (submitted)

6   Brown G, Harris T. *The Social Origins of Depression.* London: Tavistock, 1978

7   Chalder T, Power M, Wessely S. Chronic fatigue in the community: "a question of attribution". *Psychol Med* 1996; **26**: 791–800

8   Deale A, Chalder T, Wessely S. Illness beliefs and outcome in chronic fatigue syndrome: is change in causal attribution necessary for clinical improvement? *J Psychosom Res* (in press)

9   Chalder T, Wallace P, Wessely S. Self-help treatment of chronic fatigue in the community: a randomised controlled trial. *Br J Health Psychol* 1997; **2**: 189–97

10 Clements A, Sharpe M, Simkin S, *et al.* Chronic fatigue syndrome: a qualitative investigation of patients' beliefs about the illness. *J Psychosom Res* 1997; **42**: 615–24

11 Ray C, Jeffries S, Weir W. Coping with chronic fatigue syndrome: illness responses and their relationship with fatigue, functional impairment and emotional status. *Psychol Med* 1995; **25**: 937–45

12 Ware N. Society, mind and body in chronic fatigue syndrome: an anthropological view. In: Kleinman A, Straus S, eds. *Chronic Fatigue Syndrome.* Chichester: John Wiley, 1993: 62–82

13 Van Houdenhove B, Onghena P, Neerinckx E, Hellin J. Does high 'action-proneness' make people more vulnerable to chronic fatigue syndrome? A controlled psychometric study. *J Psychosom Res* 1995; **39**: 633–40

Some symptoms of CFS might suggest a cognitive impairment or organic brain disorder. Eileen Joyce describes her studies and those of others who have tested these hypotheses.

Cognitive function

Eileen Joyce

Many patients with chronic fatigue syndrome (CFS) complain not only of mental fatigue but also of poor memory and concentration. For several reasons, such cognitive complaints deserve close attention. First, the subjective perception of cognitive impairment does not necessarily signify cognitive abnormality. In various disorders with such complaints as a common factor, there is often a discrepancy between what patients report and what can be demonstrated[1]. Objective assessment is therefore important. Second, studies of cognitive function can provide clues to whether CFS has an organic aetiology. Characteristic patterns of neuropsychological impairment are associated with lesions in certain areas of the brain. For example, the amnesic syndrome, with its highly specific form of memory impairment, is caused by damage to medial temporal lobe structures or the diencephalon; and lesions of the frontal lobe produce 'executive' defects, due to the inability to optimize performance in circumstances requiring the operation of several different cognitive processes. A third reason for studying cognitive impairment is the putative link between CFS and depression. Although not all CFS sufferers are thought to be depressed[2], some researchers still speculate that the syndrome is a form of depression. Comparisons of cognitive function in depressed patients and CFS patients (with and without depressive symptoms) might help to resolve the matter.

METHODOLOGICAL ISSUES

There have been about twenty neuropsychological studies of CFS in which patients were identified according to accepted criteria and matched controls were used for comparisons (reviewed in Refs 1–3). Some investigators found no cognitive impairment, and the results obtained by others have varied greatly. One possible reason for the discrepancies is sample selection. Patients recruited in specialist settings tend to have long durations of illness, high rates of psychiatric morbidity and intense disease attributions — all of which may confound neuropsychological performance. Another possible reason is that the neuropsychological tests are not sensitive enough — because originally developed to reveal deficits in severely brain-damaged patients — or not specific for the type of cognitive abnormality characteristic of CFS. Nevertheless, some useful conclusions can be drawn from these investigations.

CONCLUSIONS FROM NEGATIVE FINDINGS

First, we can say firmly that patients with CFS do not have widespread or severe cognitive impairment. Standard intelligence tests have yielded no evidence for general intellectual decline after onset of the disorder[4-6].

A second observation is that, to date, no pattern of impairment has emerged that is either reminiscent of a brain disorder with established organic aetiology or indicative of a specific lesion of any particular brain area[7]. Although some investigators have found performance decrements on a range of neuropsychological tests, there is no evidence of a specific disorder of memory (amnesic syndrome) or frontal lobe function, or any sort of dementia. Thus, neuropsychological studies do not point to structural brain damage as the cause of cognitive complaints in CFS.

A third conclusion is that depression alone cannot account for the cognitive dysfunction in CFS. Although several research teams have found a link between objective measures of depression and aspects of cognitive performance[8-11], an equal number of others have not[4,6,7,12]. DeLuca and co-workers[13] reported that a group of CFS patients without depression were actually *more* cognitively impaired than a group of CFS patients with concurrent psychiatric disorders, most of whom were clinically depressed. Finally, Cope *et al.*[4] found no differences in cognitive performance between CFS patients with and without depression.

THE NATURE OF COGNITIVE IMPAIRMENT IN CFS

The present consensus is that objective cognitive impairments in CFS are subtle and occur when complex information processing is required[1-3]. Our own study is illustrative.

We tried to overcome the problems of sensitivity and specificity by using the CANTAB set of computerized tests[4], which have proved sensitive to mild cognitive abnormalities in psychiatric and neurological disorders and have also revealed distinct patterns of impairment in various neuropsychological conditions. We avoided selection bias by studying patients with CFS recently identified prospectively in primary care[15]. The study group consisted of 20 CFS patients and 20 controls matched for age, sex and IQ recruited from the same general practices. We employed a range of tests measuring memory, attention and executive function and the tests were graded so that we could examine the effect of cognitive fatigue on the level of achievement within each domain.

We found that the CFS patients were impaired on very few of the tests. For example, they performed normally on two complex executive tests — a test of planning and a test that measures the ability to shift the focus of attention from one stimulus dimension to another: people with frontal lobe lesions tend to score abnormally on both these tests[16–18]. They were also normal on tests of learning and recognition memory that other studies have shown sensitive to lesions of the medial temporal lobe[19], early Alzheimer's disease[20] and the amnesic syndrome[21].

Although the tests thus uncovered no impairments that might point to dysfunction of memory circuitry, we did find impairment on some measures of memory that we think can explain the subjective cognitive complaints. On a test of spatial span, CFS patients were marginally but significantly less able than controls to remember the position of a number of identical squares displayed on a computer screen. Whereas the controls could retain the position of up to six squares at once, CFS patients could only manage five. A second memory test required subjects to learn the location of nine sets of patterns individually placed in boxes on a computer screen. For each set the subject was allowed a maximum of ten trials to learn the pattern-location associations. In the first eight sets, the number of patterns presented in the boxes varied from 1 to 8. CFS patients were able to learn the location of up to 8 patterns with the same efficiency as control subjects. The ninth set also consisted of 8 patterns but, instead of the subject being reminded of the location of all patterns on each trial, only the locations of patterns incorrectly located on the previous trials were reshown. Therefore, in this selective reminding set, subjects had to maintain the memory for correctly learned pattern-location associations while learning the correct locations of patterns that they had failed to locate in the previous trial. Although the CFS subjects were eventually able to learn all pattern locations they took significantly more trials than did controls at this most effortful stage (Figure 1). Thus, both tests demonstrated subtle deficits in memory and learning: although CFS patients performed within the normal range on most memory measures they were inefficient in coping with the most difficult stages.

The most striking abnormality emerged in a test of spatial working memory. Here subjects were asked to search through a number of boxes presented on the screen to find a token. Once a token was found, that box was not used again to hide a token. The difficulty of the test could be varied by altering the number of boxes. CFS subjects made more errors than controls at the most difficult levels, showing themselves less able to keep track of the boxes that had already contained tokens while searching for new tokens (Figure 2). Further analysis revealed that the CFS group were less able to employ an efficient strategy to aid performance.

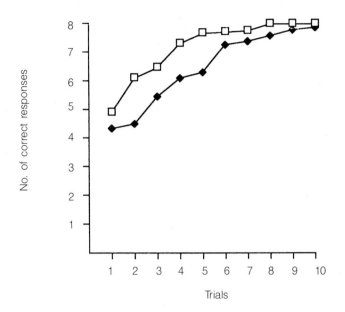

Figure 1

Number of correct pattern-location associations for each trial, selective reminding stage. (From Ref 7.) CFS, n=20; controls, n=20. □= Controls; ◆= CFS.

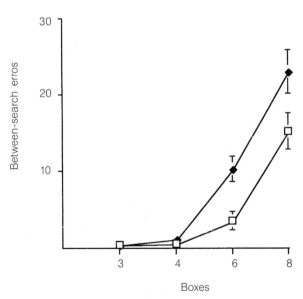

Figure 2

Errors in spatial working memory task at each level of difficulty. (From Ref 7.) CFS, n=19; controls, n=20. □= Controls; ◆= CFS.

A PSYCHOLOGICAL EXPLANATION FOR COGNITIVE DEFECTS IN CFS

A unifying explanation for our results is that, in CFS, the subjective complaints of central fatigue and of poor memory and concentration reflect a reduction of central processing capacity that can be detected objectively in effortful memory tasks. This is in line with Hasher and Zacks' hypothesis[22] that different memory tasks demand different amounts of central processing resources (or 'energy') for optimum performance. A reduction in this overall capacity will show up in performance of the most effortful tasks. According to Hasher and Zacks, the amount of processing capacity available for cognitive performance is influenced by age, by psychological factors such as arousal and mood, and by physical health — so this formulation does not help us understand why patients with CFS should have subnormal processing capacity. Wearden and Appleby[1] prefer an explanation in terms of inefficient allocation of normal processing capacity (rather than depleted capacity *per se*), to distinguish CFS from depression and to account for the discrepancy, on some memory tasks, between subjective fatigue and normal performance.

FUTURE RESEARCH

An explanation of the cognitive defects of CFS in terms of allocation of central processing may offer a useful psychological formulation but it says nothing about their neural basis. Obvious candidates are one or more of the subcortical cholinergic and monoamine neurotransmitter systems (serotonin, noradrenaline, dopamine), which in laboratory animals have been shown to mediate aspects of arousal necessary for information processing in association cortex[23]. In man, activity in these systems can be measured by several techniques including functional neuroimaging and neuroendocrine challenge tests. Future research might employ such methods in conjunction with neuropsychological tasks that specifically highlight the cognitive dysfunction we now know to exist in CFS.

REFERENCES

1 Wearden AJ, Appleby L. Research on cognitive complaints and cognitive functioning in patients with chronic fatigue syndrome (CFS): what conclusions can we draw? *J Psychosom Res* 1996; **41**: 197–211

2 Tiersky LA, Johnson SK, Lange G, *et al.* Neuropsychology of chronic fatigue syndrome: a critical review. *J Clin Exp Neuropsychol* 1997; **19**: 560–86

3 Moss-Morris R, Petrie KJ, Large RG, Kydd RR. Neuropsychological deficits in chronic fatigue syndrome: artifact or reality? *J Neurol Neurosurg Psychiatry* 1996; **60**: 474–7

4 Cope H, Pernet A, Kendall B, David A. Cognitive functioning and magnetic resonance imaging in chronic fatigue. *Br J Psychiatry* 1995; **167**: 1–9

5 DeLuca J, Johnson SK, Beldowicz D, Natelson BH. Neuropsychological impairment in chronic fatigue syndrome, multiple sclerosis and depression. *J Neurol Neurosurg Psychiatry* 1995; **58**: 38–43

6   Grafman J, Schwartz V, Dale JK, *et al.* Analysis of neuropsychological functioning in patients with chronic fatigue syndrome. *J Neurol Neurosurg Psychiatry* 1993; **56**: 684–9

7   Joyce EM, Blumenthal S, Wessely S. Memory, attention and executive function in chronic fatigue syndrome. *J Neurol Neurosurg Psychiatry* 1996; **60**: 495–503

8   McDonald E, Cope H, David A. Cognitive impairment in patients with chronic fatigue: a preliminary study. *J Neurol Neurosurg Psychiatry* 1993; **56**: 812–15

9   Krupp LB, Sliwinski M, Masur DM, *et al.* Cognitive functioning in depression in patients with chronic fatigue syndrome and multiple sclerosis. *Arch Neurol* 1994; **51**: 705–10

10 Marshall P, Forstot M, Callies A, Peterson P, Schenck CH. Cognitive slowing and working memory difficulties in chronic fatigue syndrome. *Psychosom Med* 1997; **59**: 58–66

11 Wearden AJ, Appleby L. Cognitive performance and complaints of cognitive impairment in chronic fatigue syndrome. *Psychol Med* 1997; **27**: 81–90

12 DeLuca J, Johnson SK, Ellis S, Natelson BH. Cognitive function is impaired in patients with chronic fatigue syndrome devoid of psychiatric disease. *J Neurol Neurosurg Psychiatry* 1997; **62**: 151–5

13 DeLuca J, Johnson SK, Natelson BH. Information processing efficiency in chronic fatigue syndrome and multiple sclerosis. *Arch Neurol* 1993; **50**: 301–4

14 Sahakian B, Owen A. Computerised assessment in neuropsychiatry using CANTAB. *J R Soc Med* 1992; **85**: 399–402

15 Wessely S, Chalder T, Hirsch S, *et al.* Post-infectious fatigue: a prospective cohort study in primary care. *Lancet* 1995; **345**: 1333–8

16 Shallice T. Specific impairments in planning. *Phil Trans R Soc Lond B* 1982; **298**: 199–209

17 Owen A, Downes J, Sahakian B, *et al.* Planning and spatial working memory following frontal lobe lesions in man. *Neuropsychologia* 1990; **28**: 1021–34

18 Owen AM, Roberts AC, Polken CE, *et al.* Extra-dimensional versus intra-dimensional set shifting performance following frontal lobe excisions, temporal lobe excisions or amygdalo-hippocampectomy in man. *Neuropsychologia* 1991; **29**: 991–1006

19 Owen AM, Sahakian BJ, Semple J, *et al.* Visuospatial short term recognition memory and learning after temporal lobe excisions, frontal lobe excisions or amygdalo-hippocampectomy in man. *Neuropsychologia* 1995; **33**: 1–24

20 Sahakian B, Morris R, Evenden J, *et al.* A comparative study of visuospatial memory and learning in Alzheimer-type dementia and Parkinson's disease. *Brain* 1988; **11**: 695–718

21 Joyce EM, Robbins TW. Cognitive deficits in Korsakoff and non-Korsakoff alcoholics following alcohol withdrawal and their relationship to length of abstinence. *Alcohol Alcoholism* 1993; suppl 2: 501–5

22 Hasher L, Zacks RT. Automatic and effortful processes in memory. *J Exp Psychol: Gen* 1979; **3**: 356–88

23 Robbins TW, Everitt BJ. Psychopharmacological studies of arousal and attention. In: Stahl SM, Iversen SD, Goodman EC, eds. *Cognitive Neurochemistry.* Oxford: Oxford Scientific Publications, 1987: 135–70

Thus, while there is a suggestion of subtle cognitive deficits, the aetiology of these is uncertain. Recent advances in neuroimaging technology provide several good ways to investigate brain structure and function in CFS. Tony David and Helen Cope examine the options.

Neuroimaging

Anthony S David, Helen Cope

Imaging of the brain has attracted considerable prominence in the world of chronic fatigue syndrome research. This reflects the well-justified tendency to see the main source of patients' troubles as residing in the central nervous system rather than in the peripheral nerves, muscles, or neuromuscular junction.

The first investigation with the sensitive neuroanatomical imaging technique of magnetic resonance imaging (MRI) was published by Buchwald and colleagues in 1992[1]. This study was based on what was thought at the time to be an outbreak of a chronic-fatigue-like illness associated with herpesvirus type 6 infection which occurred in the Lake Tahoe region of the southwestern United States. Multiple punctate foci of T2 high signal in the cortex and subcortical regions were reported in a very large proportion of cases (78%), compared with 21% of controls — still quite a high proportion. The findings were seen to be suggestive of central nervous system inflammation or demyelination. Critics subsequently pointed out the possibility of selection bias and misdiagnosis[2,3].

A more strictly controlled study of sporadic cases of CFS was reported by Natelson's group from New Jersey the following year[4]. In this series the frequency of subcortical hyperintensity was 27%, or 22% when they excluded 3 patients who developed other known neurological conditions. In all, 6 of 52 CFS cases versus 1 control had unexplained foci of increased white matter signal.

THE LINBURY TRUST MRI STUDY

In the study supported by the Linbury Trust[5] we sought to build on these research findings. First, a well-known association between depression and white matter hyperintensities needed to be controlled for any study of CFS, in view of the high prevalence of depression in such patients[6]. Second, the effects of viral infection needed to be taken into account, since this is thought to cause symptomless lesions. We therefore made use of an ongoing prospective study funded by the Medical Research Council, looking at new cases of post-viral fatigue[7] presenting to general practitioners in London and the South East. 26 patients who attributed their chronic fatigue to a viral illness were recruited in this way. Of this group 11 were designated as chronic fatigue, plus depression, on the basis of the caseness definition provided by the Clinical Interview Schedule and a score of >16 on the Beck Depression Inventory. These patients were compared with 18 controls who also complained to their general practitioners of having a viral infection but did not subsequently develop chronic fatigue, and, finally, a group of patients with uncomplicated depression attending the Maudsley Hospital outpatient department.

All subjects underwent a detailed neuropsychological battery as well as a thorough assessment of their symptoms of fatigue, anxiety and depression. They were scanned on a 1.5 tesla Siemen's machine and high-resolution T2 weighted images were obtained on 5 mm slices. Coronal T1 images were also obtained on 6 mm slice images. Scans were rated systematically by a consultant neuroradiologist blind to the diagnosis, and particular attention was given to the presence of deep white matter lesions as well as qualitative changes in brain morphology. The results are shown in Table 1. As can be seen, a small number of patients in all the four groups had lesions, including the control group without chronic fatigue or depression. Another observation is that depression was associated with a variety of unexplained lesions on MRI; possible explanations for this include confounding by factors such as smoking and high blood pressure. There was, however, no suggestion that chronic fatigue *per se* is associated with brain abnormalities on MRI.

Table 1. *Magnetic resonance findings in chronic fatigue, depression and normal controls* (Ref 5)

Brain region	Normal controls (n=10)	Chronic fatigue (n=13)	Chronic fatigue+ depression (n=9)	Depression (n=12)
Frontal WML	1 subject: 1 lesion (L)	1 subject: 1 lesion (L)	1 subject: 2 lesions (L+R)	1 subject: 2 lesions (L+R) 1 subject: 4 lesions (3L, 1R) 1 subject: 5 lesions (R)
Parietal WML	0	1 subject: 1 lesion (R)	1 subject: 1 lesion (R)	2 subjects: 1 lesion (R)
Total WML	1 (1 subject)	2 (1 subject)	4 (2 subjects)	12 (3 subjects)

WML=White matter lesion; L=left; R=right.

The Linbury study goes some way to exclude brain abnormalities as being relevant to the majority of sporadic cases of chronic fatigue. However, it is open to several criticisms. First, not all cases met criteria for CFS, although exclusion of patients not fulfilling the criteria did not materially alter the results. Second, the statistical power was low: at least 88 subjects, 44 cases and 44 controls, would be necessary to detect a difference between a 10% prevalence of abnormality in controls and a 20% prevalence in cases with 95% confidence and 80% power. Furthermore, the precise implications of the abnormalities detected may yet become clearer as MRI is more widely used and the range of 'normal variants' is more fully understood.

RECENT RESEARCH

A systematic literature search on neuroimaging in chronic fatigue has revealed few additional studies since the publication of the 1996 review by Cope and David[7]. One new paper, however, is important. In the study by Greco and colleagues, from University College London Medical School[8], of their 43 CFS patients, 15 had CFS by standardized criteria, 14 had CFS with depression and the remaining 14 had other non-psychotic psychiatric disorders. These had structural brain MR scanning at 1.0 tesla. The comparison group was 43 age and sex matched controls, scanned at 1.5 tesla. Abnormalities were present in 13 (32%) of the CFS group and 12 (28%) of the controls. The abnormalities were various and included areas of demyelination and single or multiple hyperintense foci in subcortical white matter structures. It should be noted that the age range of the subjects was wide — up to 78 years in the CFS group. Nevertheless, some of the younger patients had abnormal scan findings. Greco *et al.* concluded that there was no pattern of brain abnormalities specific to CFS. The study essentially replicates the Cope paper[5] and highlights the sensitivity of MR to 'abnormalities' of debatable significance.

Research interest has turned from examination of static structural brain images to dynamic neuroimaging techniques such as positron and single photon emission tomography (PET and SPET), and fMRI. These techniques display regional changes in cerebral blood flow which reflect focal brain activity. The work with SPET in CFS has been reviewed by Cope and David[3]. So far, all of it has been on resting blood flow. A wide range of abnormalities has been reported — in the main, focal areas of hypoperfusion. Interpretation is difficult because similar findings have been reported in uncomplicated depression[9]. One observation to attract considerable attention is that of brainstem hypoperfusion, reported by Costa and colleagues[10]. There are questions about the reliability of measurement of radioisotope in such a small area, since this lies at the limit of spatial resolution of the technique, and also the blindness to diagnosis of the rater;

nevertheless the findings are of interest — and will be even more so if replicated independently.

FUTURE DIRECTIONS

Although controlled structural MRI studies have not pointed to a clear excess of abnormalities in CFS patients, the matter is not completely closed since investigations to date have been on the borders of adequate statistical power. Functional neuroimaging offers more promise, especially since the waxing and waning of symptoms in CFS implies a non-structural abnormality. Resting SPET studies are of limited value, so an area that would be well worth investigation would be the use of activation techniques combined with functional neuroimaging. For example, studies of those cognitive processes prone to abnormality in chronic fatigue, such as sustained attention and working memory, could be incorporated into activation paradigms with either SPET or PET. CFS patients might be compared with psychiatric patients; or, ideally, CFS patients would be studied before and after treatment. The effects of poor performance on cerebral blood flow could be teased out by having a control group who were similarly impaired on the task, though for different reasons. If the CFS group showed specific patterns of abnormal blood flow, this would go a considerable distance in plotting a distinct neurobiological substrate for the disorder.

REFERENCES

1   Buchwald D, Cheney PR, Peterson DL, *et al.* A chronic illness characterised by fatigue, neurologic and immunologic disorders, and active human herpes type 6 infection. *Ann Intern Med* 1992; **116**: 103–13

2   Reeves WC, Pellett PE, Gary H. The chronic fatigue syndrome controversy. *Ann Intern Med* 1992; **117**: 343

3   Cope H, David AS. Neuroimaging in chronic fatigue syndrome. *J Neurol Neurosurg Psychiatry* 1996; **60**: 471–3

4   Natelson BH, Cohen JM, Brassloff I, *et al.* A controlled study of brain magnetic resonance imaging in patients with the chronic fatigue syndrome. *J Neurol Sci* 1993; **120**: 213–17

5   Cope H, Pernet A, Kendall B, David A. Cognitive functioning and magnetic resonance imaging in chronic fatigue. *Br J Psychiatry* 1995; **167**: 86–94

6   David A. The post viral fatigue syndrome and psychiatry. *Br Med Bull* 1991; **47**: 966–88

7   Cope H, David A, Pelosi A, *et al.* Predictors of chronic 'postviral' fatigue. *Lancet* 1994; **344** 864–8

8   Greco A, Tannock C, Brostoff J, Costa DC. Brain MR in chronic fatigue syndrome. *Am J Neuroradiol* 1997; **18**: 1265–9

9   George MS, Ketter TA, Post RM. SPECT and PET imaging in mood disorders. *J Clin Psychiatry* 1993; **56**(suppl): 6–12

10   Costa DC, Tannock C, Brostoff J. Brainstem perfusion is impaired in chronic fatigue syndrome. *Q J Med* 1995; **88**: 767–73

Numerous brain disorders can be linked to altered function at a neurochemical level. Tony Cleare describes progress made in defining any such disturbance in neurotransmitter function in CFS.

Neurochemistry

Anthony J Cleare

Much of the published work on chronic fatigue syndrome points to a central origin for the symptoms. Here I review research that links the syndrome with abnormalities in brain neurotransmitter systems.

SEROTONIN

Serotonin (5-hydroxytryptamine, 5-HT) has been the most studied of the central neurotransmitters. Early work in man had suggested that the fatigue felt after exercise was associated with a rise in plasma levels of tryptophan (the aminoacid precursor of 5-HT) and a reduction in other aminoacids. The effect of this would be to increase concentrations of tryptophan in the brain and thus, because the rate-limiting enzyme in 5-HT synthesis is non-saturated, raise brain 5-HT production. So it was hypothesized that high 5-HT levels could be at least partly responsible for the subjective feeling of fatigue[1]. Support for this hypothesis came from studies in which healthy subjects were given tryptophan by mouth and complained of fatigue, mental slowness and lack of vigour[2,3].

In CFS, several intriguing findings have emerged. The initial study was by Demitrack *et al.*[4], who measured 5-hydroxyindoleacetic acid (5-HIAA), the breakdown product of 5-HT, in cerebrospinal fluid and plasma as an index of the turnover of 5-HT in the brain. Concentrations were higher than in healthy controls, suggesting increased turnover of 5-HT in the brain. However, the link between these indices and brain metabolism is unclear; most of the 5-HT in plasma is of gut origin, while half of that in the cerebrospinal fluid comes from the spinal cord rather than the brain.

These observations provided the rationale for several Linbury-funded studies which set out to measure central 5-HT function more directly, by exploiting the neuroanatomical connections between the serotonergic neurons in the brainstem raphe nuclei and the hypothalamus. Release of serotonin from these projections enhances the release of hypothalamic peptides that control pituitary secretion of prolactin and corticotropin. Thus, researchers were able to administer a standardized dose of a selective drug activating elements of this pathway to obtain an overall index of 5-HT function.

Our group conducted a study with d-fenfluramine, a drug that selectively induces release of 5-HT from the raphe nuclei neurons and inhibits the reuptake of released 5-HT. We measured the endocrine responses in patients with CFS, comparing them with the responses of both healthy controls and a group of depressed subjects[5]. Although the most recent consensus criteria allow patients with co-morbid depression to receive a diagnosis of CFS, in order to get a valid comparison in this study we excluded these patients. Staff volunteers with no history of psychiatric disorder were used as controls. All participants had been medication-free for at least three months. Subjects were carefully matched for age, weight, gender and menstrual cycle. Each test involved measurement of the prolactin response to 30 mg oral d-fenfluramine over 5 hours.

The results are shown in Figure 1. CFS patients showed a distinctly higher prolactin response than controls, whereas depressed patients had a lower response. Thus, in a subgroup of non-depressed CFS subjects, we found evidence of 5-HT overactivity. The contrast with 5-HT hypofunction seen in depression suggested biological distinctions between the two syndromes, putting to rest earlier suggestions that they were one and the same. A second study with d-fenfluramine, again using non-depressed CFS subjects, confirmed this increased prolactin response[6]. A third study[7], in which the investigators used racemic fenfluramine, did not reveal any differences in prolactin responses; one possible reason is that racemic fenfluramine affects neurotransmitters other than 5-HT; another is that the investigators did not exclude CFS patients with depression.

A caveat to the method is that, if there is heightened prolactin release generally in CFS, then the results can not be interpreted as representing 5-HT dysfunction. However, our group has found that prolactin response to insulin-induced hypoglycaemia was normal or subnormal[8,9]. Thus, these results with d-fenfluramine suggest increased 'net' 5-HT functional activity, including presynaptic and postsynaptic components and all 5-HT receptors. On the hypothesis that the 5-HT1A receptor subtype is specifically affected, two groups have examined prolactin responses to the 5-HT1A partial agonist buspirone[10,11]. Both found an increased response, which they interpreted as indicating upregulated 5-HT1A receptor function. However, the results must be treated with caution because buspirone also has dopaminergic effects which could account for the prolactin response. Lastly, Dinan and co-workers used the more specific 5-HT1A agonist ipsapirone, measuring corticotropin responses[12]. These were low in CFS, but the general reduction of corticotropin response seen

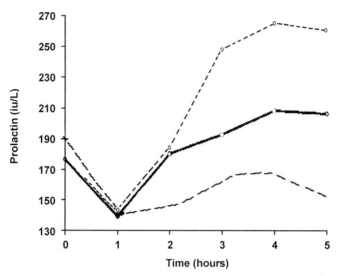

Figure 1

Mean prolactin concentrations following d-fenfluramine in patients with depression, patients with chronic fatigue syndrome, and healthy controls. - - - CFS; ——— *controls;* – – – *depression.*

in CFS suggests that this result has more to do with reduced activity of the hypothalamo-pituitary-adrenal axis than with 5-HT function (see p. 50).

In summary, most studies point to an increase in 5-HT function, and perhaps specifically of 5-HT1A receptor function. Figure 2 indicates some of the relationships. The methods for studying 5-HT function are being refined: we and others[13] have developed techniques for measuring cerebral metabolism and blood flow changes subsequent to 5-HT activation, and new receptor ligands for positron and single photon emission tomography allow quantification of receptor numbers and binding in the brain. These have already been used in depression to identify the regions of brain that possibly show subnormal 5-HT responses, and we are now trying them in CFS.

How important are these 5-HT changes in CFS? They may be of physiological significance, since 5-HT participates in the physiological control of sleep, appetite and mood. Like 5-HT, these features are disturbed in opposite directions in classic endogenous depression (insomnia, anorexia, agitation) and CFS (hypersomnia, hyperphagia and retardation). It is also conceivable that these changes are secondary to low cortisol levels[5,14,15] or the effects of inactivity, sleep disturbance or disruption of circadian rhythms. To answer some of these questions we are now assessing the effect of cortisol supplements on prolactin responses to d-fenfluramine.

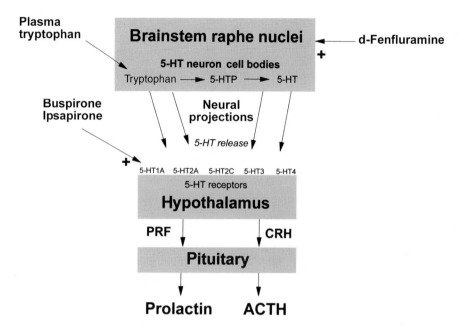

Figure 2

Schematic representation of raphe nuclei projections to hypothalamus and pituitary, indicating sites of action of drugs used in challenge studies. 5-HTP=5-hydroxytryptophan; 5-HT=5-hydroxytryptamine; PRF=prolactin releasing factor; CRH=corticotropin releasing hormone; ACTH=corticotropin.

In terms of treatment, these findings seem to favour a strategy for reducing 5-HT neurotransmission. In depression, serotonin reuptake inhibitors such as fluoxetine are able to downregulate 5-HT1A receptors; in CFS their physiological effect is not known. Research on the efficacy of such treatments has given conflicting results (see p. 63). A direct means of reducing central tryptophan, and hence 5-HT, is to administer competing aminoacids. There is experimental evidence that this strategy reduces the sensation of effort in healthy individuals[16], and in CFS some of the psychological findings, such as an enhanced sense of effort, might be linkable to these observed changes in 5-HT function.

NORADRENALINE

Studying cerebrospinal fluid and plasma in CFS, Demitrack *et al.*[4] noted low values for the main metabolite of noradrenaline, methoxyhydroxyphenylglycol. Of interest, therefore, is the study by Odagiri *et al.*[17] suggesting that fatigued athletes differed from non-fatigued athletes in having lower plasma noradrenaline. However, no other studies of noradrenergic function in CFS have been reported.

ACETYLCHOLINE

There has been one study of cholinergic function in CFS. Chaudhuri et al.[8] examined the growth hormone response to pyridostigmine, a cholinesterase inhibitor. CFS patients showed enhanced responsivity, suggesting upregulation of cholinergic receptors.

CORTICOTROPIN RELEASING HORMONE (CRH)

CRH is the neuropeptide that controls release of corticotropin from the pituitary. However, it also acts at extrahypothalamic sites as a neurotransmitter, and seems to be responsible for a syndrome of behavioural activation. Examining cerebrospinal fluid, Demitrack et al.[14] found normal amounts of CRH in CFS, though as stated earlier, these results may not accurately reflect brain levels. They did find abnormalities in the control of corticotropin and cortisol release suggestive of a deficiency of CRH at the level of the hypothalamus or above, and they offered the attractive hypothesis that a deficiency of an activating neuropeptide could contribute to fatigue. However, several of their patients were also suffering from depression. In a Linbury-funded project, our group has now replicated this study using a CRH challenge test in 36 non-depressed CFS patients and 36 controls. There were no differences in the corticotropin response to CRH — indirect evidence that CRH may not be altered in CFS[19].

CONCLUSIONS

The most compelling results from the body of work outlined is of 5-HT overactivity in CFS — in striking contrast to the picture in depression. Further work is underway with more specific techniques to assess 5-HT disturbance, to assess whether the changes are primary or secondary, and to gauge the importance of these abnormalities in relation to symptoms and possible treatments.

REFERENCES

1   Blomstrand E, Celsing F, Newsholme EA. Changes in plasma concentrations of aromatic and branched-chain amino acids during sustained exercise in man and their possible role in fatigue. *Acta Physiol Scand* 1988; **133**: 155–21

2   Greenwood MH, Lader MH, Kantameneni BD, Curzon G. The acute effects of oral (L)-tryptophan in human subjects. *Br J Clin Pharmacol* 1975; **2**: 165–72

3   Lieberman HR, Corkin S, Spring BJ, Growdon JH, Wurtman RJ. Mood, performance, and pain sensi-tivity: changes induced by food constituents. *J Psychiatr Res* 1982; **17**: 135–45

4   Demitrack M, Gold P, Dale J, et al. Plasma and cerebrospinal fluid monoamine metabolism in patients with chronic fatigue syndrome: prelimin-ary findings. *Biol Psychiatry* 1992; **32**: 1065–77

5   Cleare AJ, Bearn J, Allain T, McGregor A, Wessely S, Murray RM, O'Keane V. Contrasting neuroen-docrine responses in depression and chronic fatigue syndrome. *J Affect Disord* 1995; **35**: 283–9

6   Sharpe M, Clements A, Hawton K, *et al.* Increased prolactin response to buspirone in chronic fatigue syndrome. *J Affect Disord* 1996; **41**: 71–6

7   Yatham LN, Morehouse RL, Chisholm BT, *et al.* Neuroendocrine assessment of serotonin (5-HT) function in chronic fatigue syndrome. *Can J Psychiatry* 1995; **40**: 93–6

8   Bearn J, Allain T, Coskeran P, *et al.* Neuro-endocrine responses to d-fenfluramine and insulin-induced hypoglycemia in chronic fatigue syndrome. *Biol Psychiatry* 1995; **37**: 245–52

9   Cleare AJ, Heap E, O'Keane V, Meill J. Neuroendocrine responses to insulin induced hypoglycaemia in CFS and healthy controls. (Submitted)

10   Bakheit A, Behan P, Dinan T, Gray C, O'Keane V. Possible upregulation of hypothalamic 5 hydroxytryptamine receptors in patients with postviral fatigue syndrome. *BMJ* 1992; **304**: 1010–2

11   Sharpe M, Hawton K, Clements A, Cowen PJ. Increased brain serotonin function in men with chronic fatigue syndrome. *BMJ* 1997; **315**: 164–5

12   Dinan TG, Majeed T, Lavelle E, Scott LV, Berti C, Behan P. Blunted serotonin-mediated activation of the hypothalamic-pituitary-adrenal axis in chronic fatigue syndrome. *Psychoneuroendocrinology* 1997; **22**: 261–7

13   Mann JJ, Malone KM, Diehl DJ, Perel J, Cooper TB, Mintun MA. Demonstration in vivo of reduced serotonin responsivity in the brain of untreated depressed patients. *Am J Psychiatry* 1996; **153**: 174–82

14   Demitrack M, Dale J, Straus S, *et al.* Evidence for impaired activation of the hypothalamic-pituitary-adrenal axis in patients with chronic fatigue syndrome. *J Clin Endocrinol Metab* 1991; **73**: 1224–34

15   Scott LV, Dinan TG. Urinary free cortisol excretion in chronic fatigue syndrome, major depression and in healthy volunteers. *J Affect Disord* 1998; **47**: 49–54

16   Blomstrand E, Hassmen P, Ek S, *et al.* Influence of ingesting a solution of branched-chain amino acids on perceived exertion during exercise. *Acta Physiol Scand* 1997; **159**: 41–9

17   Odagiri Y, Shimomitsu T, Iwane H, Katsumura T. Relationships between exhaustive mood state and changes in stress hormones following an ultra-endurance race. *Int J Sports Med* 1996; **17**: 325–31

18   Chaudhuri A, Majeed T, Dinan T, Behan PO. Chronic fatigue syndrome: a disorder of central cholinergic neurotransmission. *J Chron Fatigue Synd* 1997; **3**: 3–16

The similarities between CFS and jet-lag and the effects of shift-work triggered interest in a possible disorder of circadian rhythms. Gareth Williams and Jim Waterhouse describe their hypothesis and the results of tests so far.

Circadian rhythms

Gareth Williams, Jim Waterhouse

Circadian rhythms—i.e. regular cyclic changes with a period of about a day—govern many vital functions including feeding, metabolism, the secretion of many hormones, and mood. The function of these cycles is unknown, but they evidently optimize physiological and psychological activities[1]. Individuals whose circadian rhythms are abolished or disrupted experimentally, or who are out of synchrony with the day–night cycle of their surroundings, show profound disturbances in many physiological and psychological measures[1-3]. Circumstances that disrupt circadian rhythms include experimental isolation in environments that lack any day–night cues, shift-working, and jet-lag. The consequences of circadian rhythm disturbance include not only changes in the regulation of hormone secretion and body temperature but also reductions in general wellbeing and mood, and in the ability to concentrate[1-4].

REGULATION OF CIRCADIAN RHYTHMS

Circadian rhythms consist of two components—an *exogenous* component governed by lifestyle and environment, and an *endogenous* one driven by a 'body clock'. The clock is situated in the suprachiasmatic nucleus of the hypothalamus, close to the brain centres that control body temperature, the cardiovascular system and hormone secretion.

The exogenous component depends upon the variable effects of environmental cues (*Zeitgebers*, from the German for time-giver). *Zeitgebers* include changes in light intensity through the day and night, getting up and going to bed, and normal daily routines of social interaction. The *Zeitgebers* serve to resynchronize the hypothalamic clock each day[1,5].

Many investigators of human circadian rhythms have used the cycles in core temperature and plasma levels of the hormone melatonin as markers, and the key exogenous factors that influence these two variables are the sleep/activity and light/dark cycles, respectively[6].

Healthy people show synchrony between the different rhythms and their components. Thus, evening is associated with a rise in plasma melatonin levels, due both to declining light intensity and to a clock-mediated stimulation of the pineal gland that secretes the hormone. There is also an evening fall in core temperature, mediated partly by the rise in melatonin (which opens up blood vessels in the skin, causing loss of heat), partly by the body clock itself and partly by a decline in physical and mental activity[1,5]. From these considerations it is obvious that disruption of this coordinating mechanism will have far-reaching consequences throughout the body.

HYPOTHESIS

We have investigated the hypothesis that chronic fatigue syndrome is characterized by disturbances of circadian rhythmicity, and that, at least in some patients, these circadian disturbances are responsible for perpetuating the symptoms of CFS.

There are two lines of evidence. First, the cardinal symptoms of CFS — fatigue, poor concentration, poor-quality sleep, myalgia — resemble those of conditions in which circadian rhythm is disrupted or made asynchronous with the environment; in particular, these symptoms develop in normal subjects who undertake shift-work or who are jet-lagged[1,3,7].

Second, various hormonal and other abnormalities in CFS, notably disturbed secretion of the adrenal gland, can be reproduced in healthy people by shift-working or jet-lag[8–10].

We suggested that, for some unknown reason, the circadian timing system is less effectively controlled in CFS patients, and that the reduced physical activity, lack of daily routine and social interaction and the sleep disturbances that this produces exacerbate these negative effects because of the loss of the everyday *Zeitgebers*. We further suggested that disturbances of circadian rhythm could be corrected by treatments that have been shown to resynchronize the body clock in conditions such as shift-work and jet-lag — namely, bright-light phototherapy[11,12] and melatonin administration[13].

This hypothesis and its therapeutic implications, have been explored in two studies funded by the Linbury Trust.

PILOT STUDY

In the pilot study we compared circadian rhythms in core temperature and in melatonin secretion between 15 patients with CFS and 15 healthy controls, matched for age and gender[14].

CFS was diagnosed according to standard criteria, and other causes of chronic tiredness and malaise were excluded. Core temperature was measured continuously over 24 hours with a rectal probe and a portable data logger, while melatonin secretion was measured in blood samples collected repeatedly under controlled environmental conditions between 6 pm and midnight (the time when melatonin secretion normally begins to increase[13]).

Normal subjects showed the expected relationship between the timing of the temperature cycle and the time of onset of melatonin secretion. In the CFS patients, however, this relationship was broken. We believe that this represents loss of coordination of circadian rhythmicity at a very high level.

DEFINITIVE STUDY

This study, currently in progress, aims to extend our understanding of the breakdown in circadian regulation in CFS, and to test whether bright-light phototherapy and melatonin treatment can restore normal circadian rhythms. Moreover, if our hypothesis is correct, the symptoms of CFS should improve in those patients who show improved synchrony of the circadian rhythms.

We aim to recruit a total of 50 CFS patients, including 25 with clinical evidence of depression and 25 without (this is because previous studies suggest that these subgroups may respond differently to the treatment)[9]. So far, we have recruited 41 patients from the chronic fatigue clinic at the Royal Liverpool University Hospital and a clinic at Fazakerley Hospital and by approaches to patient groups including the ME Association branches throughout Merseyside and the North-West. 32 patients remain in the study, and 3 have completed it.

As in our first study[14] circadian rhythms are being assessed from measurements of melatonin secretion and body temperature. We are also looking at the circadian rhythms in heart rate (which tends to slow during the night). The patients keep an activity diary which they fill in every half-hour during the 48-hour periods when body temperature is being monitored, and also wear a wrist 'actigraph', which records arm movements. The purpose of these two separate methods is to allow mathematical correction of the temperature recordings for physical activity, since muscle movement is thermogenic and can raise the body temperature[15].

During the study, these circadian rhythms will be examined at intervals, together with detailed scoring of the patients' symptoms, including fatigue, poor concentration, muscle aches and pains, sleep quality and depression.

The effects of *melatonin* will be investigated during these months and for a similar period the patients will receive identical placebo capsules. Melatonin will be taken at a dose of 5 mg, $2\frac{1}{2}$ hours before the median time of onset of sleep (as indicated by the sleep diary). This dosage has been found useful in jet-lag and for improving sleep quality in elderly patients; it is not associated with any important side effects.

Phototherapy is being given by seating the subject in front of a fluorescent tube unit of a type used to treat seasonal affective disorder. The patient sits down and is exposed to bright light (2500 lux) for 1 hour on rising in the morning. This schedule was chosen to regularize the patient's lifestyle; much longer exposure (up to 3 hours) is required to resynchronize circadian rhythms in conditions such as jet-lag, but we believe that the daily routine of light exposure and sitting down at a fixed time of day, together with a lesser effect of light exposure itself, will act as an effective *Zeitgeber*.

Analysis and interpretation

Patients' symptoms are being scored in a standardized and validated fashion, and the impact of melatonin and phototherapy will be assessed both in the group as a whole and in individual cases. This is because circadian rhythm disturbances may be important in causing symptoms in a specific subset, but perhaps not in all patients with symptoms that can be classified as CFS.

The measures of circadian rhythm will also be analysed to determine whether melatonin and/or phototherapy can restore the normal relation between the various rhythms.

IMPLICATIONS AND FUTURE DEVELOPMENTS

At present the aetiology of CFS is uncertain but the likelihood is that many different conditions can lead to the same symptom complex. We believe that disturbances of the coordination of circadian rhythms could be a final common pathway that might initiate and then perpetuate the symptoms, in at least a subset of patients. Disruptions of circadian rhythm could follow numerous different triggering events, ranging from intercurrent viral or other infections to episodes of depression and other adverse life events (there is a parallelism here with affective disorder).

The demonstration that the coordination of various key circadian rhythms is abnormal in CFS would have several important implications. An identifiable cause for the disease would be found, which would provide new opportunities for understanding its causes and eventual treatment. Diagnostic tests based on circadian rhythms could be developed; at present the diagnosis remains one of exclusion. Treatment of CFS might become practicable through melatonin or bright-light phototherapy or other measures that target the regulation of circadian rhythms. Pinpointing of a convincing physiological abnormality would confer medical credibility to CFS, which would become more readily accepted as a distinct medical condition by doctors and patients alike.

A note of caution

The purpose of the current studies is to test our hypothesis as rigorously as possible. We hope that melatonin or phototherapy will prove effective, but we shall not know until the results of this and perhaps other studies have been analysed in detail.

Already, however, certain medical practitioners are prescribing melatonin (not a registered drug within the UK) for people with CFS. At present we believe strongly that melatonin should be given only in the context of a controlled trial with careful analysis of physiological and symptomatic responses.

ACKNOWLEDGEMENTS
The research nurses who worked on the Linbury-funded projects were Mrs Jackie Pirmohamed, Mrs Julie Mugarza and Ms Davina Calbraith We thank our experimental subjects for committing themselves to this difficult and demanding study.

REFERENCES

1 Minors D, Waterhouse JM. Separating the endogenous and exogenous components of the circadian rhythms of body temperature during night work using some 'purification' models. *Ergonomics* 1993; **36**: 497–507

2 Folkard S. Circadian performance rhythms: some practical and theoretical implications. *Phil Trans R Soc Lond B* 1990; **327**: 543–53

3 Ross JK, Arendt J, Horne J, Haston W. Night-shift work during Antarctic winter: sleep characteristics and adaption with bright light treatment. *Physiol Behav* 1995; **57**: 1169–74

4 Van Reeth O, Sturis J, Byrne MM, *et al.* Nocturnal exercise phase delays circadian rhythms of melatonin and thyrotropin secretion in normal men. *Am J Physiol* 1994; **266**: E964–74

5 Cagnacci A, Soldani R, Yen SSC. The effect of light on core body temperature is mediated by melatonin in women. *J Clin Endocrinol Metab* 1994; **76**: 1036–8

6 Van Cauter E, Sturis J, Byrne M, *et al.* Preliminary studies on the immediate phase-shifting effects of light and exercise on the human circadian clock. *J Biol Rhythms* 1993; **8** (suppl 1): S99–108

7   Akerstedt T. Psychological and psychophysio-
     logical effects of shift work. *Scand J Work Environ
     Health* 1990; **16** (suppl 1): 67–73

8   Demitrack MA, Dale JK, Straus SE, *et al.*
     Evidence for impaired activation of the hypotha-
     lamic-pituitary-adrenal axis in patients with
     chronic fatigue syndrome. *J Clin Endocrinol Metab*
     1991; **73**: 1224–34

9   Bearn J, Wessely S. Neurobiological aspects of
     the chronic fatigue syndrome. *Eur J Clin Invest*
     1994; **24**: 79–90

10   Leese GP, Chattington PD, Fraser WD, Vora JP,
     Edwards RHT, Williams G. Short-term night-
     shift working mimics the pituitary-adrenocortical
     dysfunction in chronic fatigue syndrome. *J Clin
     Endocrinol Metab* 1996; **81**: 1867–70.

11   Terman M, Terman JS, Quitkin FM, McGrath
     PJ, Stewart JW, Rafferty B. Light therapy for
     seasonal affective disorder: a review of efficacy.
     Neuropsychopharmacology 1989; **2**: 1–22

12   Czeisler CA, Kronauer RE, Allan JS, *et al.* Bright
     light induction of strong (type 0) resetting of the
     human circadian pacemaker. *Science* 1989; **244**:
     1328–33

13   Arendt J. Mammalian pineal rhythms. *Pineal Res
     Rev* 1985; **3**: 161–213

14   Williams G, Pirmohamed J, Minors D, Waterhouse
     J, Buchan I, Arendt J, Edwards RHT. Dissociation of
     body temperature and melatonin secretion circadian
     rhythms in patients with chronic fatigue syndrome.
     Clin Physiol 1996; **16**: 327–37

16   Minors DS, Pirmohamed J, Williams G, Edwards
     R, Healy D, Waterhouse J. Circadian rhythms of
     activity and rectal temperature at home and in a
     hospital: effects of lifestyle. *Chronobiol Int* 1995;
     12: 199–205

A natural progression from abnormalities in the rhythm of hormones was to measure any changes in the hormones themselves. In particular, the possible links between CFS and stress, and the known disturbance of the main stress axis in depression, focused attention on the adrenal axis.

Neuroendocrine abnormalities: focus on the stress axis

Lucinda V Scott, Timothy G Dinan

A theoretical framework has been developed[1] that allows a conception of a variety of human disease states, cutting across psychiatric, endocrine and inflammatory disorders, based on a characteristic hyperactivity and/or hypoactivity of the generalized stress response. Corticotropin-releasing hormone (CRH) and the sympathetic nervous system are the two principal effectors of this system[2]. The stress system is switched on in response to both psychological and physical stressors. CRH activates the endocrine stress response via the hypothalamic-pituitary-adrenal axis (HPA); CRH is released from the hypothalamus, impacting at the corticotropes of the anterior pituitary and resulting in the release of adrenocorticotropic hormone (ACTH), this in turn resulting in cortisol release from the adrenal cortex.

The exploration of neuroendocrinological parameters in chronic fatigue syndrome has increased our understanding of how CFS may relate to other disorders, and in particular major depressive disorder, the differentiation of these two conditions representing one of the many contentious issues in CFS research. Though depressed mood is present in most patients with CFS[3,4], the general view is that they represent two overlapping but distinct conditions[5]. Studies to date do not support the notion that concurrent depression in a person with CFS is simply a reaction to the disability itself[4].

The evidence for a dysregulated HPA system in major depression began with Gibbons and McHugh's demonstration of elevated baseline cortisol levels[6]. We now know that many patients with major depression are dexamethasone non-suppressors[7], have a blunted ACTH response to CRH administration[8], have enlarged adrenal glands[9] and have an exaggerated response to stimulation with exogenous ACTH[10].

HPA FUNCTION IN CFS

The evidence that HPA activity is dysregulated in depression, coupled with the symptomatic overlap between CFS and glucocorticoid insufficiency, provided ample reason for an exploration of HPA function in CFS; the paper of Demitrack and colleagues[11] provided the first assessment of HPA activity in this disorder. Basal cortisol and ACTH levels were examined, as were 24-hour urinary free cortisol (UFC) levels, plasma cortisol binding globulin (CBG) and cortisol responses to graded stimulatory doses of exogenous ACTH. 30 subjects with CFS, diagnosed according to CDC criteria, and 72 healthy controls took part in this series of investigations. Low basal cortisol levels, high basal evening ACTH levels, normal levels of CBG and low 24-hour UFC levels were found, together with blunted ACTH release in response to a standard CRH infusion and enhanced response to low-dose infusion.

We too have found a low 24-hour UFC in chronic fatigue syndrome[12]. We compared 15 CFS subjects (CDC criteria) with 15 healthy subjects and 11 subjects with DSMIIIR major depression. All participants were medication-free for 4 weeks before the study. The depression group had 24-hour UFC values significantly higher than the other groups, with values in the healthy subjects intermediate. Of further note was the fact that the 3 CFS patients who had a co-morbid major depression retained the UFC profile of those with CFS alone. This observation adds to evidence that the two conditions are endocrinologically distinct, and also suggests that when the two disorders are concurrent the biological profile of CFS overrides that of the depressive disorder. Larger studies are required.

Demitrack's demonstration of low basal cortisol levels[11] has not been so readily replicated. Although Cleare and co-workers[13] did find lower basal cortisol concentrations in CFS subjects (CDC criteria) than in healthy and depressed cohorts (the latter having higher basal cortisol values than either of the others), negative results have been obtained in several other studies[14–17]. The discordance may reflect methodological differences across studies, most notably variations in sampling times, but principally it serves to highlight the weakness of a single cortisol measurement as an indicator of overall HPA activity. Work by our group points also to a defect at adrenal androgen level; dehydroepiandrosterone (DHEA) and DHEA-sulphate (DHEA-S) were lower in CFS than in healthy subjects, whereas only DHEA-S was lower in a depressed cohort[18]. The deficiency of DHEA and DHEA-S in CFS patients points to inadequate neurotropic stimulation at adrenocortical level.

INTEGRATION

To integrate these findings, a theory of mild central adrenal insufficiency has been proposed[11]. This model is attractive since chronically low cortisol levels provide an acceptable explanation for some of the more non-specific findings of immune activation in CFS, such as raised viral antibody titres and increased allergic sensitivity. Supportive evidence for this proposal has accumulated. Using a low-dose (1 μg) ACTH test, an examination of adrenocortical function regarded as more 'physiological' than the standard 250 μg version, we demonstrated blunted release of cortisol in CFS compared with that in healthy subjects[16]. This was interpreted as an indication of reduced adrenal secretory reserve, due to inadequate stimulation either from pituitary or central level. We also administered 100 μg ovine CRH and found release of ACTH, and of cortisol, to be attenuated in non-depressed CFS subjects compared with healthy volunteers[17]. Further support for the above interpretation was our demonstration, in a preliminary computer tomography study, of smaller adrenal glands in CFS patients who had biochemical evidence of low adrenocortical output[18].

Together with CRH, arginine vasopressin (AVP) is a key regulator of HPA activity and becomes increasingly so in situations of stress[19]. In patients with CFS we co-administered CRH and dd-AVP and compared the response with that to CRH administered on its own[20]. While CFS subjects showed the typical blunted response to CRH alone, the response to the combination was indistinguishable between CFS patients and controls. This raises the possibility of enhanced vasopressinergic activity in CFS.

Defective activation of the pituitary-adrenal system in CFS has not been shown by the insulin hypoglycaemia test, generally regarded as the gold standard of HPA activators. Bearn and colleagues[14] found no difference between CFS patients and healthy subjects in ACTH or cortisol response to insulin challenge, but did find significantly lower prolactin responses and a trend towards lower concentrations of growth hormone. An exaggerated ACTH response but normal cortisol response to d-fenfluramine challenge — a test that provides an index of serotonergic mediated HPA activation — did support a theory of altered adrenocortical functioning and fuelled the possibility that dysregulated HPA activity may be serotonergically mediated (see p. 38).

Dinan et al.[21] investigated the above possibility by stimulating the HPA with ipsapirone, the 5HT1a partial agonist, and significant attenuation of ACTH release in CFS patients relative to healthy controls provided support for the view that serotonin is involved in the pathophysiology of CFS[22]. A low opioid tone might explain the multiple somatic symptoms such as muscle and joint pain experienced by CFS patients. Scott et al.[23] gave naloxone (the opioid antagonist) to CFS patients and healthy subjects and found a decreased release of ACTH in CFS, suggesting low opioid tone.

Overall, the studies to date indicate that patients with CFS have abnormalities in the HPA, probably due to decreased central drive. Further work needs to focus on the reasons for such disturbance — and in particular whether the described anomalies are primary, or secondary to decreased activity.

REFERENCES

1 Chrousos GP, Gold PW. The concepts of stress and stress system disorders. *JAMA* 1992; **267**: 1244–52

2 Gold PW, Goodwin F, Chrousos GP. Clinical and biochemical manifestations of depression: relationship to the neurobiology of stress, Part 1. *N Engl J Med* **319**: 348–53

3 Manu P, Lane TJ, Matthews DA. The frequency of chronic fatigue syndrome in patients who complain of persistent fatigue. *Ann Intern Med* 1988; **109**: 544–6

4 Wessely S, Powell R. Fatigue syndromes: a comparison of chronic 'postviral fatigue' with neuromuscular and affective disorders. *J Neurol Neurosurg Psychiatry* 1989; **42**: 940–8

5 Demitrack MA. Neuroendocrine correlates of chronic fatigue syndrome: a brief review. *J Psychiatr Res* 1997; **31**: 69–82

6 Gibbons J, McHugh P. Plasma cortisol in depressive illness. *Psychiatr Res* 1963; **1**: 162–71

7 Carroll BJ, Curtis GC, Mendels M. Cerebrospinal fluid and plasma free cortisol concentrations in depression. *Psychol Med* 1976; **6**: 235–44

8 Holsboer F, Von Bardeleben U, Wiedemann K, *et al.* Blunted corticotropin and normal cortisol response to human corticotropin-releasing factor (h-CRF) in depression. *N Engl J Med* 1984; **311**: 1127

9 Rubin R, Philips J. Adrenal gland volume in major depressives. *Arch Gen Psychiatry* 1993 **50**: 833–4

10 Amsterdam J, Winokur A, Abelman E, *et al.* CoSyntropin (ACTH 1-24) stimulation test in depressed patients and healthy subjects. *Am J Psychiatry* 1983; **140**: 907–9

11 Demitrack MA, Dale JK, Straus SE, *et al.* Evidence of impaired activation of the hypothalamic-pituitary-adrenal axis in chronic fatigue syndrome. *J Clin Endocrinol Metab* 1991; **73**: 1224–34

12 Scott LV, Dinan TG. Urinary free cortisol excretion in chronic fatigue syndrome, in depression and in health. *J Affect Disorders* 1997; **47**: 49–54

13 Cleare AJ, Bearn J, Allain T, *et al.* Contrasting neuroendocrine responses in depression and chronic fatigue syndrome. *J Affect Disorders* 1995; **34**: 283–9

14 Bearn J, Allain T, Coskeran P, *et al.* Neuroendocrine responses to d-fenfluramine and insulin hypoglycaemia in chronic fatigue syndrome. *Biol Psychiatry* 1995; **37**: 245–52

15 Yatham LN, Morehouse RL, Chisholm BT, *et al.* Neuroendocrine assessment of serotonin (5HT) function in chronic fatigue syndrome. *Can J Psychiatry* 1995; **40**: 93–6

16 Scott LV, Medbak S, Dinan TG. The low dose adrenocorticotropin test in chronic fatigue syndrome and in health. *Clin Endocrinol* (in press)

17 Scott LV, Medbak S, Dinan TG. Blunted adrenocorticotropin and cortisol response to corticotropin releasing hormone stimulation in chronic fatigue syndrome. *Acta Psychiatr Scand* (in press)

18 Scott LV, Teh J, Reznek R, Sohaib A, Dinan TG. Small adrenal glands in chronic fatigue syndrome: a preliminary computer tomography study. (Submitted)

19   Saillard R, Riondal A, Ling N, Muller A. Corticotropin-releasing factor activity of CRF41 in normal man is potentiated by angiotensin II and vasopressin but not by desmopressin. *Life Sci* 1988; **43**: 1935–44

20   Scott LV, Medbak S, Dinan TG. Evidence for increased anterior pituitary vasopressinergic responsivity in chronic fatigue syndrome. (Submitted)

21   Dinan TG, Majeed T, Lavell E, *et al*. Blunted serotonin-mediated activation of the hypo-thalamic-pituitary-adrenal axis in chronic fatigue syndrome. *Psychoneuroendocrinology* 1997; **22**: 261–7

22   Bakheit AM, Behan PO, Dinan TG, *et al*. Possible upregulation of 5-hydroxytryptamine receptors in patients with post-viral fatigue syndrome. *BMJ* 1992; **304**: 1010–12

23   Scott LV, Medbak S, Dinan TG. Blunted naloxone mediated ACTH release in chronic fatigue syndrome. *Psychol Med* 1998 **28**: 285–92

TREATMENT

Numerous treatments for CFS have been suggested or piloted in open uncontrolled studies but few have been subjected to the rigorous methodology of the randomized controlled trial. Three treatments are described in this section, all tested in more than one such trial. Peter White describes the results with graded exercise.

Graded exercise therapy

Peter White

People with chronic fatigue syndrome are less active than healthy people. We should not be surprised that tests of aerobic capacity show them to be less physically fit[1], since rest leads to physical deconditioning. Would they be helped if they could regain their fitness? In fibromyalgia, a condition that overlaps with CFS[2], fitness training was more effective than flexibility exercises, not only in improving aerobic capacity but also in reducing muscle pain[3]. The Linbury Trust funded two projects to test the hypothesis that graded exercise therapy is useful in CFS.

THE BART'S TRIAL

In the first study, at St Bartholomew's Hospital and the National Sports Medicine Institute, Kathy Fulcher and I compared graded aerobic exercise with flexibility and relaxation treatment[4]. Before the main study, we excluded (or alternatively treated) patients with psychiatric illnesses such as depressive illness and a small number of patients who had serious insomnia. We did this because sleep disturbances and depressive illness can by themselves cause excessive fatigue. 167 patients were screened and 96 patients were excluded, most commonly because of a depressive illness. Treatment of depressive illness usually alleviated fatigue to the extent that patients no longer met criteria for the study. 71 patients were offered entry into the study: 5 patients declined and 66 agreed.

Patients were randomly allocated to one or other treatment and were seen weekly for twelve weeks, with equal therapist time for either treatment. Those in the graded exercise group were given their own exercise programme, designed for their current level of activity. They were encouraged to exercise five days a week, but the initial sessions lasted only about ten minutes, giving an intensity of exercise which put their heart rate up only moderately. A heart rate monitor was used to make sure they reached but did not exceed their target heart rate; this boosted patients' confidence that they were not overdoing things. At each weekly meeting they increased their daily exercise prescription by one or two minutes, up to a maximum of thirty minutes a day. Once at that exercise duration they increased the intensity of the exercise. Exercises included walking as well as cycling and swimming. If fatigue became more severe with the treatment, they were advised to stay at the same level of exercise for longer rather than increasing it, until they had adapted to the higher exercise level.

Few patients dropped out of either treatment. 16 of 29 (55%) of those who completed twelve weeks of graded exercise treatment rated themselves as 'much better' or 'very much better' than before the treatment started. This contrasted with 8 of 30 (27%) who rated themselves better after flexibility treatment—a significant difference. Only 1 in each group felt worse after completing treatment. When the results were analysed according to 'intention to treat' (to allow for the drop-outs), the difference between treatments was still significant. Of those who completed the flexibility treatment, 22 of the original 33 went on to graded exercise therapy. Three months after stopping supervised graded exercise treatment, 32 (68%) of 47 patients who attended follow-up rated themselves as better; and after a year 35 (74%) of 47. Fatigue, physical capacity, fitness and muscle strength all improved significantly with graded exercise therapy. By a year of follow-up, two-thirds of patients were working or studying at least part-time. Although complete recovery was rare, clinically important effects on both symptoms and disability were recorded in most of the patients.

A detailed description of graded exercise therapy has now been published, so that others can apply it[5].

THE MANCHESTER TRIAL

Alison Wearden and colleagues[6], from Manchester, examined the effects of both graded exercise therapy and the antidepressant fluoxetine in a randomized controlled trial (see p. 63). The effect of graded exercise therapy was less impressive than that observed in the Bart's study: although completed exercise treatment improved fatigue and aerobic work capacity at both 12 and 26 weeks, there was no significant effect on perceived disability. 18% of patients receiving exercise treatment were no longer 'cases' of CFS by 26 weeks, compared with 6% of those treated without exercise. Fluoxetine had no significant effects on fatigue, anxiety or aerobic capacity, but did improve depression. In this study about one-third of patients dropped out of graded exercise therapy before completing the course and a further third did not adequately adhere to the prescribed exercise. On analysis of the data by intention to treat, the significant effect on aerobic capacity persisted but there was only a trend for less fatigue, at twelve and twenty-six weeks.

SUCCESS AND FAILURE

Why were the Manchester results less impressive than those of the Bart's study? 46% of Wearden and colleagues' patients had a psychiatric illness (mainly depressive illness) and some had major sleep disturbances; these features, in themselves predisposing to fatigue[7–9], might have reduced the efficacy of graded exercise. Interestingly, the patients with depressive illness tended to find graded exercise helpful only if they also received the antidepressant. Another difference between the trials was that in the first twelve weeks the Manchester therapists saw the patients 5 times compared with 12 times at Bart's, started exercise treatment at a more intense level and increased intensity only when the patients had shown physiological conditioning. Neither trial indicated that graded exercise was harmful, which is a natural fear of sufferers. Both support the suggestion that 'rest has no place in treating chronic fatigue'[10].

Why did graded exercise therapy help when it did? There are several possibilities. Although improved fitness and muscle strength can be expected to lessen fatigue, the Bart's trial showed that such improvements do not correlate with 'feeling better'. Patients are wary of exercise treatments, often because a previous exercise programme has failed. Understandably, they lose confidence in their ability to undertake any serious exercise; but if we expose them to exercise in a controlled way they regain confidence in their bodies and become more active, with the attendant physiological benefits of that activity.

Why do some exercise programmes *not* work? Sleep disturbance and psychological distress, with their independent effects on fatigue[7,8], may need treatment in their own right, with the later addition of exercise treatment if necessary. The way graded exercise treatment is given may also influence the outcome.

NEXT STEPS FOR RESEARCH

Answers to the following questions would be valuable. Are the Bart's and Manchester findings replicable in different samples and centres? How does graded exercise therapy compare with cognitive behaviour therapy? Can we predict who will respond to graded exercise therapy and who to cognitive behaviour therapy? How can sufferers be more easily engaged in graded exercise therapy? In depressive illness non-aerobic exercise therapy is no less effective than aerobic[11]: will this be true in CFS? How will group treatment compare with individual treatment?

REFERENCES

1   Saltin B, Blomquist G, Mitchell J, *et al*. Response to exercise after bedrest and after training. *Circulation* 1968; **38**(suppl 7): 1–55

2   Buchwald D, Garrity D. Comparison of patients with chronic fatigue syndrome, fibromyalgia, and multiple chemical sensitivities. *Arch Intern Med* 1994; **154**: 2049–53

3   McCain GA, Bell DA, Mai FM, Halliday PD. A controlled study of the effects of a supervised cardiovascular fitness training program on the manifestations of primary fibromyalgia. *Arthritis Rheum* 1988; **31**: 1135–41

4   Fulcher KY, White PD. Randomised controlled trial of graded exercise in patients with the chronic fatigue syndrome. *BMJ* 1997; **314**: 1647–52

5   Fulcher KY, White PD. Chronic fatigue syndrome: a description of graded exercise treatment. *Physiotherapy* (in press)

6   Wearden AJ, Morriss RK, Mullis R, *et al*. A randomised, double-blind, placebo controlled treatment trial of fluoxetine and a graded exercise programme for chronic fatigue syndrome. *Br J Psychiatry* 1998; **172**: 485–90

7   Myles WS. Sleep deprivation, physical fatigue, and the perception of exercise intensity. *Med Sci Sports Exercise* 1985; **17**: 580–4

8   Morgan WP. Psychological components of effort sense. *Med Sci Sports Exercise* 1994; **26** 1071–7

9   Royal Colleges. *Chronic Fatigue Syndrome: Report of a Joint Working Group of the Royal Colleges of Physicians, Psychiatrists and General Practitioners*. London: Royal College of Physicians, 1996

10 Sharpe M, Wessely S. Putting the rest cure to rest—again. *BMJ* 1998; **316**: 796

11 Martinsen EW. Therapeutic implications of exercise for clinically anxious and depressed patients. *Int J Sport Psychol* 1993; **24**: 185–99

Cognitive behaviour therapy begins with a cautious exploration of the role of conscious beliefs in determining behaviours. It then proceeds to a series of behavioural experiments aimed at reducing the inconsistent activity patterns characteristic of CFS, and subsequently to a gradual reduction of avoidances and an increase in activity. Michael Sharpe describes the results.

Cognitive behaviour therapy

Michael Sharpe

Cognitive behaviour therapy (CBT) is a practical, non-pharmacological, approach to treatment of chronic fatigue syndrome. It offers patients a new way to think about their illness and to cope with it that in turn allows them to achieve improvements in their functioning. With its combined approach of talking, record keeping and patient-monitored increases in activity, CBT overlaps substantially with some exercise programmes [1,2].

The first application of CBT to chronic fatigue syndrome was by Wessely and colleagues, working at a hospital for neurological disorders in London. Proposing a vicious-circle model of the perpetuation of chronic fatigue whereby patients' beliefs about the illness led to avoidance of activity and thus to chronic disability, they found that a graded approach to rehabilitation could greatly improve the functioning of hitherto bedbound patients; these benefits were, by and large, maintained at follow-up[3,4].

A COGNITIVE BEHAVIOURAL MODEL OF CFS

The initial attempt at treatment was thus promising, and challenged the therapeutic nihilism prevalent at that time. Our group wanted to develop the behavioural approach, and the first step was to interview 66 CFS patients in depth so as to gain a systematic view of their beliefs and behaviour. On qualitative analysis we found that most patients saw themselves as helpless to overcome the physical disease process that (they believed) underlay their fatigue; all they could do for their symptoms was to rest or keep activity to a minimum[5]. We proposed a detailed cognitive behavioural model of CFS whereby patients' experience of the illness shaped such beliefs, which in turn drove avoidance behaviour (either continuous or intermittent) and perpetuated the condition[6].

RANDOMIZED TRIALS OF CBT

With this deeper understanding of patient's beliefs about their illness we elaborated a form of CBT that focused on beliefs as well as behaviour. Would this variant of CBT be more effective than non-specific medical management in patients with disabling CFS? A group of us, then based in Oxford, randomized 60 patients to either sixteen sessions of CBT or to ordinary medical care[7]. At the final outcome assessment (twelve months after randomization and eight months after the end of treatment) about two-thirds of the patients who had received CBT were functioning at a satisfactory level, compared with only a quarter who had been given ordinary medical care. The CBT group also reported less fatigue.

This result was encouraging. But did the benefit simply reflect the time we had spent with these patients? The group from King's College Hospital, London, conducted a further trial of this form of CBT using a similar design, except that they compared CBT with a similar number of sessions of relaxation therapy — to determine whether the results of the first trial had simply reflected the effect of spending time with this neglected patient group. The observed benefit of CBT was similar to that obtained in the first trial, and the effect of relaxation was little different from that we had obtained with ordinary medical care. CBT therefore seemed to have a specific beneficial effect in many patients with CFS.

MECHANISM OF ACTION

CBT as given in the trials described above is a complex treatment. It helps patients to re-evaluate their beliefs, encourages them to change their behaviour and also fosters a problem-solving approach to social and occupational difficulties. Which of these is the active ingredient — or are all necessary?

There were two main ways to address this question. First we could look at process measures and see which variables change in patients who improve with treatment. Both the above trials incorporated a simple measure of the belief that 'exercise is harmful', and this belief was abandoned by a greater proportion of those who received CBT — evidence that change in the belief is an important factor in recovery. Second we could 'dismantle' the therapy and determine the effectiveness of single components. This alternative approach was tried by a group from St Bartholomew's Hospital, London, who assessed a behavioural treatment of highly supervised graded increases in activity (without specific cognitive or problem-solving components) by comparison with flexibility exercises[1]. They found that patients improved more with graded exercise. Does this finding mean that a behavioural therapy of increased activity is all that is needed? Perhaps not, because the patients were a selected group and also received detailed explanation from the exercise therapist. Indeed a further trial from Manchester, evaluating a less intensively supervised exercise regimen in unselected referrals, seemed to confirm the need for a cognitive component in the therapy: many patients declined to participate in the treatment and many others dropped out from exercise—presumably because they did not believe it was helpful[2].

LONG-TERM OUTCOME OF CBT

We were also interested to know just how long the benefits of CBT lasted, especially since the limited follow-up data suggested that patients continued to improve over the eight months after the four months of therapy had ended. Preliminary results from long-term follow-up of the first randomized trial[7] show that, although many patients maintain their improvement, a proportion 'slip back'. Perhaps active follow-up, with 'booster' sessions, would help maintain improvement. Further studies are required to evaluate such strategies.

CBT AND THE BIOLOGY OF CFS

The trials of CBT have shown that 'psychological' treatment is effective in patients with CFS. Does that mean that it is 'all in the mind'. As reviewed elsewhere in this publication, there are measurable abnormalities in the brains of at least some patients with CFS—in the serotonergic neurotransmitter system, for example[8,9] (see p. 38). One way to determine whether such abnormalities are causally associated with the symptoms and disability of CFS would be to see how they change with response to treatment. This has not yet been done.

CBT AS A DELIVERABLE TREATMENT

Treatment with CBT requires a skilled therapist—and few such therapists are available. We may therefore wonder whether it could be delivered by a nurse, or even in self-help form? Studies are now being conducted to address these questions. Already there is evidence that a self-help book coupled with a single session from a nurse is helpful to patients with fatigue in primary care[10]. The development of a form of CBT that is both effective and readily delivered throughout the National Health Service remains an important challenge.

CONCLUSIONS

Cognitive behaviour therapy is currently the most effective treatment we have for CFS but it is rarely curative and does not work for all patients. We do not fully understand the mechanism of action: it seems to include changes in both behaviour and belief. Important outstanding questions about CFS include the following. Can we make the therapy more effective so that it helps a greater proportion of patients? Can we clarify its mechanism of action, especially in terms of biology? Can we devise an effective form of CBT that can be administered by relatively unskilled persons, or even as self-help?

REFERENCES

1   Fulcher KY, White PD. A randomized controlled trial of graded exercise in patients with the chronic fatigue syndrome. *BMJ* 1997; **314**: 1674–52

2   Wearden A, Morriss RK, Mullis R, *et al*. A double blind, placebo controlled trial of fluoxetine and a graded exercise programme for chronic fatigue syndrome. *Br J Psychiatry* 1998; **172**: 485–90

3   Wessely S, David AS, Butler S, Chalder T. Management of chronic (post-viral) fatigue syndrome. *J R Coll Gen Practit* 1989; **39**: 26–9

4   Bonner D, Ron M, Chalder T, Wessely S. Chronic fatigue syndrome: a follow up study. *J Neurol Neurosurg Psychiatry* 1994; **57**: 617–21

5   Clements A, Sharpe M, Borrill J, Hawton KE. Illness beliefs of patients with chronic fatigue syndrome: a qualitative investigation. *J Psychosom Res* 1997; **42**: 615–24

6   Surawy C, Hackmann A, Hawton KE, Sharpe M. Chronic fatigue syndrome: a cognitive approach. *Behav Res Ther* 1995; **33**(5): 535–44

7   Sharpe M, Hawton KE, Simkin S, Surawy C, Hackmann A, Limes I, Peto T, Warrell D, Seagroatt V. Cognitive behaviour therapy for the chronic fatigue syndrome: a randomized controlled trial. *BMJ* 1996; **312**: 22–6

8   Sharpe M, Clements A, Hawton KE, Young AH, Sargent P, Cowen PJ. Increased prolactin response to buspirone in chronic fatigue syndrome. *J Affect Disord* 1996; **41**: 71–6

9   Sharpe M, Hawton KE, Clements A, Cowen PJ. Increased brain serotonin function in men with chronic fatigue syndrome. *BMJ* 1997; **315**: 164–5

10 Chalder T, Wallace P, Wessely S. Self-help treatment of chronic fatigue in the community: a randomized controlled trial. *Br J Health Psychol* 1997; **2**: 189–97

A large proportion of CFS patients fulfil diagnostic criteria for both CFS and depression, and many clinicians resort to antidepressants for treatment. Alison Wearden and Louis Appleby review the results of the surprisingly few clinical trials published to date.

Antidepressant therapy

Alison Wearden, Louis Appleby

Many symptoms of chronic fatigue syndrome overlap with those of depressive disorders. Fatigue, sleep disturbance (including sleeping too much), difficulties with concentration and memory, and depressed mood are common to both. When 'co-morbid' psychiatric disorders have been sought in CFS patients, depression has been found in as many as 54% — even when fatigue was excluded from the diagnostic criteria for depression[1].

Is the depression a non-specific response to chronic illness, or is it part of the CFS symptom complex? One observation favouring the latter is that depression is more common in CFS than in other fatiguing illnesses with comparable disability. Another is that the symptom profile of depression in CFS may be subtly different from that in primary depression, with a lower rate of depressive cognitions such as suicidal ideas[2,3]. Yet another is that CFS and depression seem to be endocrinologically distinct[4,5] (see p. 50).

Lynch and co-workers[6] have argued that, no matter what our concept of depression in CFS, we ought to treat if symptomatically with antidepressants. First, however, we need to know whether antidepressants are tolerated by CFS patients and whether they are effective against depression in this group. Other important research issues are whether antidepressants improve other symptoms of CFS, particularly fatigue, and whether they work equally well in CFS patients with and without depression.

CLINICAL EXPERIENCE AND OPEN TRIALS

Several groups have claimed clinical success in treating the mood symptoms of CFS[6-8]. Because tricyclic antidepressants have sedative effects, most have opted to use monoamine oxidase inhibitors (MAOIs) or selective serotonin reuptake inhibitors (SSRIs). Behan and colleagues[9] reported an open uncontrolled study of the SSRI sertraline, administered for six months at a dose of 50 mg per day. Sertraline was well tolerated and most of the patients improved in terms of fatigue, muscle pain, sleep disturbance and depression. The presence of symptoms of depression at initial assessment had no effect on outcome (although none of them had had major depression at that time).

In another open uncontrolled study, White and Cleary[10] used the MAOI moclobemide 600 mg daily in CFS patients. After six weeks' treatment 50% of those who had initially been depressed rated themselves better overall, compared with only 19% of non-depressed — 19% being about the proportion one would expect to benefit from a placebo. Moclobemide was well tolerated, only 8% of patients dropping out of treatment because of side-effects.

DOUBLE BLIND PLACEBO-CONTROLLED STUDIES

Clinical observations and open studies may provide useful hints, but proof of clinical efficacy requires double-blind trials. The evidence so far is meagre. In a small randomized trial, Natelson and colleagues[11] administered low doses of the MAOI phenelzine or placebo over six weeks with a two-week placebo run-in phase. Although drug-treated patients showed improvement over a wider range of assessments than placebo-treated patients, the two groups did not differ on any individual outcome variable, including the measure of depression. 3 of 15 patients (20%) stopped taking phenelzine before completing the six weeks of treatment.

Vercoulen et al.[12] compared the SSRI fluoxetine 20 mg daily with placebo in 96 patients. After eight weeks' treatment they found no difference between drug and placebo on any of a range of outcome measures, including depression (not even in CFS patients with a concurrent diagnosis of depression). Surprisingly, there was no evident placebo effect on any of the measures. Fluoxetine was only moderately well tolerated: 15% of drug-treated patients stopped treatment because of side-effects compared with 4% of those taking placebo.

In our Manchester study[13] we used the same dose of fluoxetine but gave it for six months and included a graded exercise programme in the comparison. 136 patients fulfilling the Oxford criteria for CFS[14] were randomly assigned to one of four treatment groups — namely, fluoxetine and a graded exercise programme; fluoxetine and appointments only; the graded exercise programme; and placebo drug. We assessed exercise capacity and measured improvement in terms of changes on a fatigue scale[15], the Medical Outcomes Survey (MOS) Short Form scales[16] and the Hospital Anxiety and Depression (HAD) scales[17]. 30 patients dropped out before completing six months' treatment — 13% of those assigned to fluoxetine and 3% of the placebo group because of medication side-effects (Table 1). Unlike Vercoulen et al.[12], we saw improvements on all measures during the course of the trial, whether patients were allocated to active or placebo treatments. Fluoxetine was more effective than placebo drug in reducing HAD scores at three months but not at six months. 46 (34%) of our patients

Table 1 *Medication side-effects that caused patients to drop out of treatment*

	Fluoxetine (9 drop-outs)	Placebo (2 drop-outs)
Nausea	3	1
Tremor, agitation	2	1
Rash	2	0
Sleep disturbance	2	0
Weight loss	1	0

One patient taking fluoxetine withdrew because of more than one side-effect.

had depressive disorders at the outset. After six months, depressed patients allocated to fluoxetine showed a greater improvement in HAD scores than non-depressed patients; however, a similar, although smaller, difference was seen between depressed and non-depressed patients allocated to placebo. Fluoxetine did not significantly affect fatigue, anxiety, exercise capacity, or any of the MOS scale scores. We found no interactions between the effects of fluoxetine and those of exercise.

CONCLUSIONS

Ours is the first controlled study to provide support, albeit modest, for the use of fluoxetine in CFS with depression. We had a large number of dropouts, many of them for reasons other than medication side-effects, and for purposes of analysis we had to record these patients as unchanged; this weakness might have obscured some of the benefit from fluoxetine, and the study requires replication.

Where do we now stand with antidepressants in the treatment of CFS? The clinical indications for these drugs remain uncertain. Possible subjects for research are whether treatment works best if started early; whether improvement of mood in the early stages has additional benefits in the long term; whether different antidepressants, or the same ones in different doses, have more powerful effects; whether best results are obtained with combinations of treatment. We also need to know more about predictors of treatment response. Larger, preferably collaborative, studies may provide the answers.

REFERENCES

1   David AS. Postviral fatigue syndrome and psychiatry. *Br Med Bull* 1991; **47**: 966–88

2   Powell R, Dolan R, Wessely S. Attributions and self-esteem in depression and chronic fatigue syndrome. *J Psychosomat Res* 1990; **34**: 665–73

3   Johnson SK, DeLuca J, Natelson BH. Depression in fatiguing illness: comparing patients with chronic fatigue syndrome, multiple sclerosis and depression. *J Affect Disord* 1996; **39**: 21–30

4   Cleare AJ, Bearn J, Allain T, *et al.* Contrasting neuroendocrine responses in depression and

chronic fatigue syndrome. *J Affect Disord* 1995; **35**: 283–9

5   Strickland P, Morris R, Wearden A, Deakin B. A comparison of salivary cortisol in chronic fatigue syndrome, community depression and healthy controls. *J Affect Disord* 1998; **47**: 191–4

6   Lynch S, Seth R, Montgomery S. Antidepressant therapy in the chronic fatigue syndrome. *Br J Gen Pract* 1991; **41**: 339–42

7   Butler S, Chalder T, Ron M, Wessely S. Cognitive behaviour therapy in chronic fatigue syndrome. *J Neurol Neurosurg Psychiatry* 1991; **54**: 153–8

8   Wilson A, Hickie I, Lloyd A, Wakefield D. The treatment of chronic fatigue syndrome: science and speculation. *Am J Med* 1994; **96**: 544–50

9   Behan PO, Haniffah BAG, Doogan DP, Loudon M. A pilot study of sertraline for the treatment of chronic fatigue syndrome. *Clin Inf Dis* 1994; **18**(suppl): S111

10 White PD, Cleary KJ. An open study of the efficacy and adverse effects of moclobemide in patients with the chronic fatigue syndrome. *Int Clin Psychopharmacol* 1997; **12**: 47–52

11 Natelson BH, Cheu J, Pareja J, *et al.* Randomised, double-blind, controlled placebo-phase-in trial of low dose phenelzine in the chronic fatigue syndrome. *Psychopharmacology* 1996; **124**: 226–30

12 Vercoulen JHMM, Swanink CMA, Zitman FG, *et al.* Randomised, double blind, placebo-controlled study of fluoxetine in chronic fatigue syndrome. *Lancet* 1996; **347**: 858–61

13 Wearden AJ, Morris RK, Mullis R, Strickland PL, Pearson DJ, Appleby L, Campbell IT, Morris JA. A randomised, double-blind, placebo controlled treatment trial of fluoxetine and a graded exercise programme in chronic fatigue syndrome. *Br J Psychiatry* 1998; **172**: 485–90

14 Sharpe MC, Archard LC, Banatvala JE, *et al.* A report — chronic fatigue syndrome: guidelines for research. *J R Soc Med* 1991; **84**: 118–21

15 Chalder T, Berelowitz G, Pawlikowska T, *et al.* Development of a fatigue scale. *J Psychosomat Res* 1993; **37**: 147–53

16 Stewart AL, Hays RD, Ware JE. The Medical Outcomes Survey Short-form General Health Survey: reliability and validity in a patient population. *Med Care* 1988; **26**: 724–34

17 Zigmond AS, Snaith RP. The Hospital Anxiety and Depression Scale (HAD). *Acta Psychiatr Scand* 1983; **67**: 361–70

EDITORIAL AFTERWORD

The decade since Holmes and co-workers made their case definition of chronic fatigue syndrome has been a time of remarkable progress. In the UK, Linbury-funded work has contributed greatly to this research enterprise. From existing evidence we can state confidently that CFS is a symptom complex rather than a disease; it is multifactorial in origin; it is not an inflammation of brain or a muscle disease; it is not solely depression; it accounts for a substantial burden of illness within the community. Numerous psychological and physiological disturbances have been identified, but large gaps in our knowledge remain. What sort of people are most likely to get it, and when? What perpetuates disability? What is cause and what is effect? How should CFS be prevented and treated?

As an editor, I have seldom encountered a set of typescripts with more 'buts'. Apart from the conflicting data, the whole area is beset with uncertainties about what is primary and what is secondary. Seeking enlightenment, I asked Dr Tony Cleare (Linbury Research Fellow) to attempt a diagrammatic synthesis of the phenomena reviewed in this booklet. He produced the figure on the next page, from which the vast potential for further research immediately becomes apparent—at levels from consulting-room to molecular laboratory.

In view of these opportunities, has the time come for a drive to defeat CFS in the next decade? Such a campaign would doubtless be as futile as the American effort to 'conquer cancer in the 1970s'. The important thing is that good ideas attract funding, and that advances in knowledge are communicated to practitioners and patients. Contributors to this booklet have offered their own research proposals; and, for separation of cause and effect, many of these would best be explored in multidisciplinary projects that draw upon prospective community-based studies. The simplest strategy, though arduous enough, is to select just one of the high-risk events from the top right-hand corner of Cleare's schema and examine its impact in a defined population—on variables ranging from the rate of sick-note writing to the sensitivity of central 5-HT receptors. Linbury-funded groups have already done work of this sort on Epstein–Barr virus and other viral infections as they arise within the community. Such investigations will not, of course, tell us about the natural history of the syndrome as a whole; and to determine this we need a large prospective investigation, which might perhaps be tacked onto one of the national epidemiological projects.

What about treatment and prevention? This booklet deals only with graduated exercise, cognitive behaviour therapy and antidepressants, but other possible strategies (including homoeopathy) are waiting in the wings. Though the results in the first two are particularly

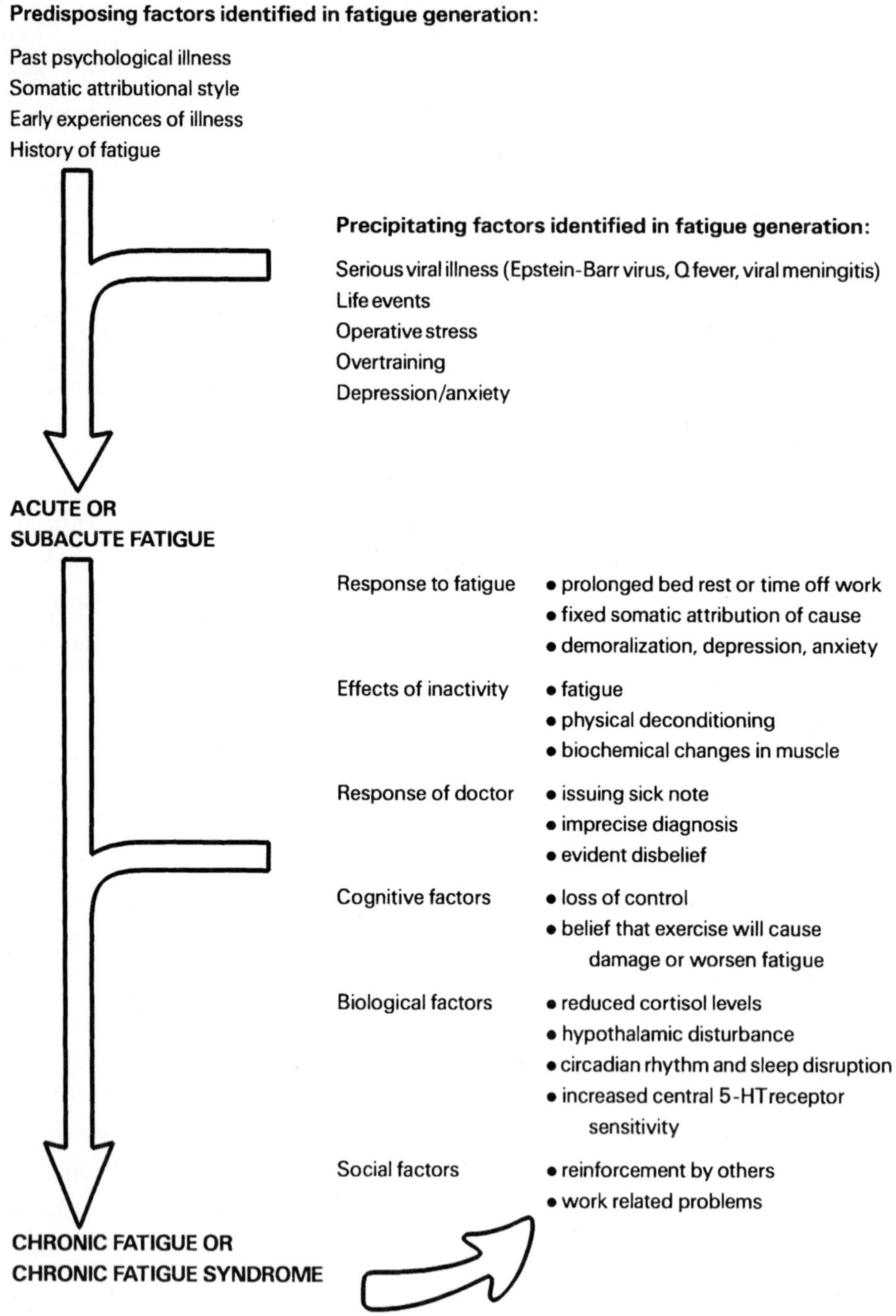

Predisposing factors identified in fatigue generation:

Past psychological illness
Somatic attributional style
Early experiences of illness
History of fatigue

Precipitating factors identified in fatigue generation:

Serious viral illness (Epstein-Barr virus, Q fever, viral meningitis)
Life events
Operative stress
Overtraining
Depression/anxiety

**ACUTE OR
SUBACUTE FATIGUE**

Response to fatigue	• prolonged bed rest or time off work
	• fixed somatic attribution of cause
	• demoralization, depression, anxiety
Effects of inactivity	• fatigue
	• physical deconditioning
	• biochemical changes in muscle
Response of doctor	• issuing sick note
	• imprecise diagnosis
	• evident disbelief
Cognitive factors	• loss of control
	• belief that exercise will cause damage or worsen fatigue
Biological factors	• reduced cortisol levels
	• hypothalamic disturbance
	• circadian rhythm and sleep disruption
	• increased central 5-HT receptor sensitivity
Social factors	• reinforcement by others
	• work related problems

**CHRONIC FATIGUE OR
CHRONIC FATIGUE SYNDROME**

Figure 1

Cleare's schema: there will be much interaction between factors.

encouraging, these treatments are time-consuming and expensive and we would be unwise to recommend them without knowing their feasibility and effectiveness in wider practice. As to prevention, one of the most intriguing observations concerns the effect of medical behaviour (and the interventions of other interested groups) on the course of the illness. In designing trials, we must not forget the possibility that some interventions will do harm; and an important yield of research might be information on what *not* to say and do when a person comes to the surgery with a complaint of fatigue.

Some of the strongest complaints about the medical profession concern the management of chronic illness. What Linbury has begun with CFS should now be pursued by larger funding bodies. An expansion of the work could illuminate large areas of medical practice that at present lie beyond the reach of evidence-based medicine.

APPENDIX

Linbury Trust

Projects at 1 June 1998

1 Charing Cross Hospital, London
1990–94
An epidemiological study into the incidence and nature of CFS
Dr D J M Wright

2 Rayne Institute, St Thomas' Hospital, London
1990–94
Research into the effects of viral infection of neuro-transmitters and the possible reversal of these effects with antidepressant drugs
Professor H E Webb

3 Institute of Psychiatry and Institute of Neurology, London
1991–94
Cognitive functioning and magnetic resonance imaging in CFS
Dr Helen Cope

4 Brunel University, Uxbridge, and Royal Free Hospital, London
1991–92
Variability in symptoms in patients with CFS
Dr Colette Ray

5 University of Oxford
1993–95
Sleep, neurotransmitter function and fatigue in patients with CFS
Dr Michael Sharpe

6 King's College Hospital and Institute of Psychiatry, London
1991–93
Hypothalamopituitary function in CFS
Dr Jenny Beam

7 St Bartholomew's Hospital and the London Sports Medicine Institute, London
1991–93
Activity level and physiological response to activity in CFS; a randomised controlled study of graded exercise programme for patients with CFS
Dr P D White

8 St Bartholomew's Hospital, London
1993
T-cell subsets in post-viral fatigue syndrome
Dr P D White

9 University of Manchester
1992–94
A double-blind placebo controlled trial of aerobic rehabilitation and fluoxetine in CFS
Dr Louis Appleby

10 University of Liverpool
1992–94
A study of the molecular mechanisms that mediate tissue adaptation in CFS
Professor M J Jackson

11 University of Oxford
1992–94
A study of the role of aminoacids in CFS
Dr E A Newsholme

12 St Mary's Hospital Medical School, London
1992–94
A study of the persistence of enteroviruses in post-viral fatigue syndrome
Professor J F Mowbray

13 Ruchill Hospital, Glasgow
1992–95
Molecular analysis of polymerase chain reaction products homologous to enteroviral sequences derived from CFS
Dr G B Clements

14 University of Bristol
1992–95
The role of psychosocial factors and recurrent infection in the pathogenesis and treatment of CFS
Professor A Smith

15 University of Liverpool
1993–95
*Circadian rhythmicity and sleep disturbance in CFS:
effects of bright light photo-therapy and dothiepin
treatment*
Professor G Williams

16 Institute of Psychiatry, London, and Queen
Mary's University Hospital, Roehampton
1992–94
*The neuropsychological basis of central fatigue in the
post infectious fatigue syndrome*
Professor Simon Wessely

17 University of Aberdeen Medical School
1992–95
Virus-induced dysfunction during ME/CFS
Dr Phillip Cash

18 London Homoeopathic Clinic
1993–94
*An investigation into the efficacy of homoeopathic drugs
in the treatment of post-viral fatigue syndrome*
Mr Richard Awdry

19 St Bartholomew's Hospital, London
1995–96
*Ambulatory study of activity and physiological response
to activity in patients with CFS*
Dr P D White

20 University of Oxford
1994–95
*Sleep disorders and their relation to daytime problems
in children with CFS*
Dr Gregory Stores

21 Charing Cross and Westminster Medical School,
London
1994–96
*A multidisciplinary study into the incidence and nature
of post-infectious fatigue syndrome*
Dr D J M Wright

22 Coppetts Wood Hospital
1994–97
*A study of the immunology, virology and therapy in
CFS*
Dr Barbara Bannister

23 University of Toronto
1994–
*A chronobiological study of sleep-immune-neuroendocrine
functions in CFS*
Dr Harvey Moldofsky

24 University College, Galway
1994–96
*Molecular analysis of HLA type in CFS: search for a
pattern of genetic inheritance*
Dr E J Fitzgibbon

25 University of Wales College of Medicine, Cardiff
1995–97
*Examination of enteroviral exacerbation of symptoms
in CFS following oral polio virus vaccination, linkage
to shedding, mutation and specific immunological
responses*
Professor Andrew Smith

26 Addenbrooke's NHS Trust, Cambridge, and
King's College School of Medicine, London
1995–97
*An investigation of neuroendocrine and serotonin
abnormalities in CFS*
Dr Veronica O'Keene

27 Lewisham and Guy's Mental Health NHS Trust,
London
1995–96
Investigation of pineal melatonin secretion in CFS
Dr Theodore Soutzos

28 St Mary's Hospital Medical School, London
1996–97
Children and adolescents with CFS: a follow-up study
Professor Elena Garalda

29 Ruchill Hospital, Glasgow
1996–
*Further characterisation of enteroviral sequences found
in patients with CFS: prospective follow up of a cohort
of patients*
Dr G B Clements

30 St Bartholomew's and The Royal London School
of Medicine and Dentistry, London
1996–97
*Regulation of HPA axis in CFS: a study in feedback
mechanisms and adrenal gland volume*
Professor Ted Dinan

31 University of Manchester
1996–97
A pilot study of a new instrument to measure family responses to CFS
Dr Louis Appleby

32 University of Aberdeen
1996–97
Defective leukocyte interactions in CFS
Dr Phillip Cash

33 University of Liverpool
1996–97
Investigation and treatment of circadian rhythm disorders in CFS
Professor Gareth Williams

34 University of Wales College of Medicine, Cardiff
1996–97
A study of enterovirus infections in patients with CFS
Dr Julie Fox

35 University of Oxford
1996–97
Cognitive behaviour therapy for CFS patients: a long-term follow-up
Dr Michael Sharpe

36 University of Glasgow
1996–
Molecular characterisation of the mechanics of enteroviral persistence and elucidation of the role of enterovirus in CFS
Dr J W Gow

37 University of Hertford
1996–97
To design a homoeopathic trial in the treatment of CFS
Dr Elaine Weatherley-Jones

38 University of Liverpool
1996–
An evaluation of different methods of challenging illness beliefs in the treatment of CFS
Professor R P Bentall

39 Guy's and St Thomas' Medical and Dental School, London
1997–98
Neurohypophyseal function in patients with CFS
Professor M Forsling

40 King's College School of Medicine and Dentistry and the Institute of Psychiatry, London
1997–
Investigation of 5-HT and hypothalamopituitary function in CFS using neuroendocrine and neuroimaging techniques
Dr A J Cleare

41 Imperial College School of Medicine at St Mary's, London
1997–
The nature and specificity of fatigue syndromes in childhood and adolescence
Professor M E Garralda

42 University of Oxford
1997–
5-HT2C receptor function in CFS
Professor P J Cowen

43 University of Sheffield
1997–
Efficacy of homoeopathic treatment for CFS patients
Dr Elaine Weatherley-Jones

44 University of Bristol and University of Wales
1998–
Viral infection and CFS
Dr Julie Fox

45 King's College School of Medicine and Dentistry, London
1998–
Antibodies to nuclear envelope antigens in CFS
Dr M Peakman

46 University of Oxford
1998–
Aminoacids and 5-HT in fatigue and immunosuppression: overtraining as a model for CFS
Dr Linda Castell

47 Guy's and St Thomas' Medical and Dental School, London
1998–
Randomized controlled trial of the equivalence of graded exercise versus cognitive behaviour therapy for patients with fatigue in general practice
Dr Leone Ridsdale